HAVING HEALTHY HAIR AT HOME

You can have it too!

PAMELA FREDERICK MAIR

Purpose Publishing
1503 Main Street #168 • Grandview, Missouri
www.purposepublishing.com

ISBN: 978-0692710029

Editing by Rosalind Bauchum
Book Cover Design by PP Team of Designers

All scripture contained in this book are referenced from the King James, New King James Versions.

Printed in the United States of America

This book is not intended as a substitute for the medical advice of physicians. The reader should regularly consult a physician in matters relating to his/her health and particularly with respect to any symptoms that may require diagnosis or medical attention.

DEDICATION

To the Creator of Heaven and Earth, the one Who was in the beginning and was with GOD, to the One who made all things, and without Him nothing would have been made. In Him is life, and He is the light for all mankind. He also became flesh, and walked among men, to the One who furnished us with the ability to use His creation, and on the third day created herbs, and vegetation for the healing of the nations. To "El Hayyay," the GOD of my Life for all His provisions, I say Thank You!

This is my first written, and printed project to manifest. I dedicate this book to the one whom I left my mother and father to cleave. After twenty-eight years of working through the madness; two becoming one flesh, and after all the "I need to understand you, so you can understand me," we did it! Honey we made it! We still have ample time to become better and closer! My husband I love you, Lij M. Mair.

Your patience with me has matured far more than what I could have ever have expected, your love for me is truly unconditional and your wisdom is clearly from our Abba Father God! I love you without measure or waiver, it is my prayer and heart's desire that you fulfill all the dreams and goals you carry deep within your heart. You deserve it! You Are worth it! Together with Christ as our guide, let's keep reaching for the stars and beyond!

To my children, I love you both Vonnie and Pops, may favor with GOD and man and all who may come in contact with you. My prayer is for God to continue to follow you and overtake all of your days for the rest of your lives. To my grandbabies, C. I. M. and our newest addition, MuMu. Grandma is glad you are both on the earth to do great and marvelous things for the kingdom of GOD.

Finally, to all my Kitchen Beauticians striving for an alternative way to care for your hair, enjoy learning and gleaning from off the pages of this book, keep learning and don't stop here, there is more out there. Keep an open mind remember more and IS NOT better nor is it faster. With discipline wisdom understanding and knowledge you will reach your goal in "Having Healthy Hair @ Home!

FOREWORD

Having Healthy Hair at Home: A Holistic Approach

PASTOR BILLY THOMPSON, SR.

I remember the first time I heard Pam speak about healthy hair. This was no ordinary conversation as she spoke with such passion and authority on health, hair and holistic approaches to improve the quality of life. My wife and I were so blown away and impressed with her depth of knowledge that we had to invest in her products. Our hair improved and so did our confidence in knowing we had someone who knew what she was talking about!

Our crash course on healthy hair which included subjects like why hair breaks off, greys early and falls out left me feeling as though we had encountered a real-life scientist! Needless to say, Pam's years of research has led her to create products containing natural herbs and oils which counteract the negative effects of the chemicals which destroy hair. Her approach to healthy hair care is one that can be embraced by everyone. I believe that you will benefit greatly from the practical solutions and suggestions contained within these pages. Not only will you see tremors results, but you will feel better from the inside out. My wife and I did!

Billy Thompson
Senior Pastor- JP Proclaim Int'l
Former NBA- Los Angeles Lakers/Miami Heat

CONTENTS

FROM THE AUTHOR

Genesis 1:11 And God said, Let the earth bring forth grass, the herb yielding seed, and the fruit tree yielding fruit after his kind, whose seed is in itself, upon the earth: and it was so.

Genesis 1:12 And the earth brought forth grass, and herb yielding seed after his kind, and the tree yielding fruit, whose seed was in itself, after his kind: and God saw that it was good. KJV

Pamela Frederick Mair is the Owner, CEO and Founder of Rxestoratives Hair and Skin Wellness®, Inc. Where she is a Holistic Cosmetologist, Hair Health Educator, Nutritional Consultant and the manufacturer of an all natural hair & skin product line. It's her mission to teach consumers how to have "Healthy Hair at Home." As a Licensed Holistic Hair Care Specialist, Cosmetologist, and a Nutritional Consultant, Pamela is committed to providing a safe, supportive and empowering environment best suited for your hair, body and skin care needs. Pamela offers Holistic Nutritional Consultations and Seminars with insightful guidance to gain a deeper understanding of how to maintain optimal health and vitality for your hair, body and skin.

It's her belief that "what goes in is what comes out!". Once the consumer has a full understanding of this concept of healing, health and wellness, restoration is within reach.

She creates a proven effective holistic hair and skin plan according to your specific needs and goals. She states, "Our body has the God given natural ability to heal itself" –in which she strongly believes. She provides gentle guidance and holistic consultations to aid in the healing restorative process whether it's for your body or the health of your hair and skin.

Nutrition is one of the key factors to attaining optimal overall health and through a verbal, visual evaluation and/or a written assessment of your current diet and lifestyle, a nutritional program can be tailored to meet your specific needs. It's her goal for you to construct a healthier, happier, and balanced life for optimal health, beautiful skin and to have stronger longer thicker hair. At her practice, she has the ability to manufacture specific all natural products just for you that will facilitate transformation to a healthy overall lifestyle.

With a full understanding and knowledge of the proper use of products, knowing what type of product is needed & having a full understanding of the "HOW TO's" as it pertains to hair/skin products, food, supplements and vitamins -YOU CAN HAVE HEALTHY HAIR AT HOME!

CHAPTER 1

My Holistic Hair Journey

My journey starts out like most hair disaster stories I have heard over the years. I am now a licensed Holistic Cosmetologist, Certified Nutritional Consultant, & certifying other stylist to become a Certified Holistic Hair Care Specialist.

Life is worth living especially when you understand the purpose of living or merely existing. I am the second oldest in my family and the eldest daughter, once my parents had two additional girls four and six years later, hair care became my primary job. As my sisters grew older, I was glad to take care of their hair. I thought this would help my mother as she worked as a nurse. In addition, providing hair care for my sisters would allow my sisters to feel good about themselves as young ladies. Hair styles and the right attitude is essential no matter the age of the person.

The years passed and time went on, but I continued to provide my sisters and my mother's hair care until a year ago, (2015) I thoroughly enjoyed doing their hair especially after I started creating my own hair and skin products. My family became my instant Ginny-pigs. This is where the Holistic journey begins:

In 1998, I decided to color my hair blonde. As a natural redhead, all my life, the color was boring to me. Not that I needed any excitement in my life but that's another book within itself; but red hair was old and played out for me. Plus, everyone was dying their hair blonde, why not join in on that action. I went to the "hair store" nit knowing what to purchase or buy. I asked the lady behind the counter (like we all are guilty of doing- so don't judge me) "what do I use to dye my hair blonde?" The attendant looked at me strangely noticing my "natural red hair," Finally she said, "oh you could use '***THIS,***" referring to white powder bleach with 40 volume! This suggestion seemed to imply I knew what to do with this product and how to use it!

I returned home to start the process of "transitioning to blonde!" I Received a phone call from one of my sisters; the one who you just can't say "Hi; and how are you? Ok, you are good, great, BYE! No not this one sister; she goes on and on and wait one more thing, oh; I forgot to tell you this, Hold on I must tell you one more thing -then "I'm a let you go!" My sister; I love her to pieces though! While we were talking, I began to smell ammonia. I said to her, "girl hold on, I think the children are in the bathroom playing in ammonia!" When I rushed to the bathroom to fuss at the children, I realized no one was in the bathroom! My hair was completely full of ***whitestuff***! I forgot I was bleaching my hair! I rushed to the tub and began to rinse my hair. While I'm rinsing the bleach out, I suddenly realized I am rinsing my hair out as well! Not knowing what the damage was I proceeded with caution as I finished washing my hair. My husband came home later that night gave me one look, and shook his head. I was a stay at home mom who was very creative, very busy, constantly doing and trying new things. He never knew from week to week what he was coming home to. One week I painted the bedroom turquoise, and purple then another week I made our bed into a canopy type bed. Another time I painted fish on the walls. Consequently, this crazy hair didn't surprise him at all.

Days went by and I began to get depressed. My hair was damaged and I didn't know what to do. I went to Bible study one Wednesday night and our pastor was teaching on *"asking God for what we want, however, we must believe when asking the Father."* We must believe that He is able to do whatsoever we ask, as long as we believe in our heart, He will be faithful to grant us our prayer. "*Whatsoever ye shall ask the Father in my name, he will give it you*". (King James Version). I prayed, "Lord, please help me, and give me directions as to what to do with my hair." This was my prayer, a whatsoever prayer asking God to please show me how to restore my hair, my thought was since chemicals took my hair out, I wanted something natural to regrow to restore my hair. Not fully understanding what natural was, I knew within myself I didn't want to use any chemicals. I was too embarrassed to go to a salon and tell respond to question of "*what had happened.*"

A few days later I was at my mother's house. My mother was a LPN nursing instructor at one of the vocational schools in Dade County, Florida. Someone gave my mother a thick book with 972 pages. Mom said, "Pam one of my students gave me this book; if you want it you can have it." The book had very few pictures in it. I took the book and looked through it and thought; who would sit down and write this many pages with hardly any relevant pictures in it? I begin to flip through the book to see what was in it. I found the most interesting ***things*** in this book. There were things (I had to call it ***things*** because at this moment in time I was ignorant regarding herbs). This book had information that advised you on how to treat high blood pressure, headaches, muscle spasms, gout, fever, diabetes, swollen limbs, bleeding open cuts, gingivitis, just anything that pertained to the body. Realizing this was the answer to my Whatsoever prayer…☺ I flipped to the back of the book to look up hair and what did I find, information in the book about hair! There were twenty different pages on herbs to take, things to do, remedies to apply yes, all of that and more. Now my brain was about to explode- and I thought; where can I get these ***items?*** Uhmmm let me see; Oh, I got it, I can call 411.

Anyone born before 1985 knows about 411 and the "411 operators." I thought to myself, "I can call the operator and ask her for information." I did need some information. When the operator answered the phone the first question was, “What city and state?”, ‘what listing?’ After remembering the routine of 411 I said, “ok here goes nothing.” I dialed 411, the operator asked. “what city and state?” “Well,” I replied, “I’m in Miami, so Miami. “What listing,” “Well” I said, “I need help with this.” The operator says “ok let's go, what is it?” I said “Well, I need lavender, sage, basil, chamomile, and burdock root.” The operator responded, says “oh it sounds like you need a vitamin store.” I said, “Yes! Sure! Ok!”. Now anyone who remembers 411 already know if you didn’t have the city and state, or the listing; just forget it! The operator stayed on the phone with me and went through all the listings from southwest Miami to where I lived in the Aventura and 163rd Street area. We even covered the area within ten miles of my residence. She located a vitamin shop on 163rd street and I said “Yes! Yes! Yes! that is close enough, thank you! Yes! give me that number” which, she did.

I immediately called the vitamin shop. The gentleman who answered the phone said; “good afternoon this is Barry, how may I help you?” I immediately blurted, “do you have Burdock Root, Nettle, Horsetail, Coltsfoot, and Spearmint?” He says, “wow sounds like you are in need of hair care herbs!” I said yes, “I am!” He replied “well I’ve got it, so come on in!” I said, “I’ll be there within fifteen minutes!” Once I arrived at the store, I was there for over three hours with him.

I thank God for Barry. He took his time and explained every herb there was for hair and scalp. Just like the information in the book; he talked about the purpose of herbs, how to use them, how to blend them, and how to apply them. I was in heaven! The more he spoke, the more I begin to feel like I can do this! I can grow my hair back with these herbs! After three hours and $200 dollars later, I went home and my journey began with a holistic outlook on life, and a new perspective pertaining to hair care.

I rushed home to start my re-growing process. I grabbed a big stock pot, filled it with water, and poured all the herbs I bought from Barry. I let the pot cool down, and scooped out the mixture and put it in my hair. Barry told me everything! One thing he forgot to tell me was I would need help which my husband provided to me later that night.

My husband came home and on that what did he find? My head full of herbs, twigs, sticks and leaves. He just dropped his head and said, "come on let me help you." He sat with me and plucked out all the herbs, twigs, sticks, and leaves. My four and seven-year-old children told their dad, "Mommie has been in the jungle and it's all in her hair!" After we finished this task my husband showed me how to handle fresh herbs. My husband is Jamaican and I'm American. I knew nothing about tea, the only thing I knew to do with tea was to drink it! I knew about sweet tea from a local fast-food restaurant. We reheated the concoction and let it cool. Next after he strained and cooled the mixture, we noticed this clear oil on top and some gooey stuff on the bottom.

Lij then said to me, "maybe you should use this," and I did. I grabbed a glob of this gooey stuff put it all over my hair, and I did this for a few weeks. I begin to do research on all the herbs I put in that pot. Several weeks went by and all I was doing was reading, studying, with a lot of research. I read everything and anything on herbs, essential oils, damaged hair, over processed hair, and whatever I could find on treating hair.

I begin to purchase the herbs in bulk and study them further, this went on for over a year. I needed to know more about these herbs and how they make the hair grow. With reading, studying and praying the entire time, began to hear formulas: sage, nettle, coconut oil. I wrote down what I'd just heard during prayer time, I researched, reviewed, and determined what this formula would be beneficial for. Through following the Holy Spirit, I learned how to utilize the herbs, and how I should apply them to the hair. I learned how to apply liquids, a butter, or a rinse and the application of various formulas on the hair. After hearing additional formulas, I would say to myself, "oh, this is for hair loss" or "oh, that formula is for dandruff." This catapulted me into the world of manufacturing all natural products. My first product was Tress Pomade.

When using my formulas on my hair, people started asking me; "what are you using in your hair?" I told them this all natural product I mixed. Several people wanted the products and I gave it to them. After applying products to their hair, users began to noticing a change in their hair. I gained new customers who wanted to come over to get their hair done. Now, my husband would come home to a house full of hair and ladies. One night, I guess he had enough. He came home and said "that's it! He continued to yell; "you! you! And you! Get out! "Come out of me house!" He's Jamaican so you know how that goes at times.

Soon after, another year had passed and by this time I knew it was time to do something different. I went to cosmetology school. Even at cosmetology school I earned hair service credits by teaching the class. Instead of doing the hair services for credit, *(but please don't tell anyone this*) I would teach the teacher and the class interesting facts about herbs, and hair and how they relate. If I think about it, this is what I'm doing now- teaching stylist in how to become a Holistic Hair Care Specialist. I am teaching you about herbs and their benefit as it pertains to hair care and *How to Have Healthy Hair at Home*. Months passed and I graduated from Cosmetology school with a small cliental and several natural hair care products.

For me it was time to take this to the next level. Still spending time in prayer, and in my books gaining more of an understanding of herbs essential oils, butters, clays only expanded. Now I am mixing and making all type of natural products especially for people who needed something when they had tried everything.

Next level was to do a seminar but the only dilemma I faced was my speech. From the age of 8 I begin to stutter due to a traumatic situation in my life. And then two more similar situations happened that followed at the age of 13, then again at the age of 16. Consequently, talking to people was not my strong point especially a group of people and especially in public.

I recall one time I was at a fast food restaurant famous sandwich with cheese, extra mayo cut in half sandwich. I would have to write my order down or have someone else place the order for me and the drive thru for me was out. Thank God I had children. My daughter from the age of five would have to place the order for me. This one day I went in to order my food and thought I can do this! I can place the order without writing it down! I waited for the line to empty, then I approached the counter. The girl greeted me as usual; "welcome and may I take your order?" I opened my mouth to place the order and nothing would come out but stuttering wha-wha-wha-wha! I told myself to take a breath, let's start over "may I have a wh-wh-wh-wh-wh-wh." "Ok Pam, I'm telling myself, calm down, breathe, and start over. "Yes, can I have a wha-whaa-whaaaa-whaa-wha-wh", nothing is coming out but these annoying sounds. The words are literally stuck in my throat, and refusing to come out. Then all of a sudden, the girl asked the man behind me, yes behind me, now there is a line about five people looking at me crazy. She asks him, "Sir may I take your order?" I said very loudly; "take his order, what do you mean take his order! Don't you see me standing here giving you my order, and you are just going to overlook me and say, "sir, may I take your order?" No! No! You will not take his order because I'm giving you my order! No one is giving any orders until I'm finish giving my order! now you all understand that! Now back to you Miss, "Can I have a wha-whaa-whaaaa-whaa-wha-whaaa, give me a pen and some paper so I can write my order down!"

This was a day I'll never forget. This is a funny story when I tell it during my seminars, and its funny just reflecting on it now. But back to my story;

Once while preparing for a seminar, I scheduled a hotel in Miami Lakes. I met with my sisters, and asked them to help me at the seminar. They both agreed to help. In my head, helping meant to do the talking for me. I met with them and explained everything, I begin to drill the information in them so they would know everything about the products. From the beginning, my sisters knew what the products were for and how they helped people with different hair and scalp issues. However, they both said "NO!" Both told me, "this is your product line, you have the passion for this, and we will not do this for you." See I could talk with my sisters without stuttering without problems; but talking to other people was a major issue for me. The day of the seminar I set up the conference room, and went out to another room to finish getting ready. At show time, I entered the room and oh boy it was full, nearly 87 people showed up to my first seminar! Even through the fear of speaking, I spoke the best I could, I would stammer at times but by the grace of GOD I told myself, "I can do all things through Christ who strengthens me." I even had to say out loud at times during the seminar to help me through some of the challenging parts of stuttering, but overall it went very well! I was so proud of myself, and I thanked GOD for the courage He gave me to do this seminar, and many other seminars that followed.

In dealing with this speech impediment I had to search deep within myself to find out why am I still stuttering after so many years since these traumatic events has happened. Soon after this heart to heart I had with myself, we were celebrating Thanksgiving with our family, and one of my relatives approached me in front of everyone to apologize for what had happened to me years earlier. I dropped my head in shame at first, but then realized this was a genuine apology, now it was up me to hold on to it or to forgive and let go. I chose to forgive and let go and almost as soon as I released them from this tragedy my speech began to clear up. ***Forgiveness is powerful tool.*** Now people meet me and would never know I had a speech impediment when I was younger.

I look forward to doing seminars and presentations with no hesitation. Now looking back at the product line, each product has its own unique story.

A lot of people ask me at my seminars how do I come up with these formulas and the best way for me to explain it is this way. "Do you know when you are driving on the highway, and "something tells you to exit," but you don't exit, and because of traffic you may end up sitting on the highway for over an hour? Then you tell yourself "something told me to exit!" Well that is how I hear formulas, this 'something' that told you to exit, and you clearly heard it tell you to do something. This is the same "something" that tells me or gives me formulas. I called that something the Holy Spirit speaking within me, directing me, and leading me into all truths (which are the formulas). He wants the best for us, He doesn't want us sitting in traffic jams or ending up in bad situations so that 'something' gives you an unction to protect you and He is here to keep us safe and protected. And when we listen **every time** we would never be in a "bad regretful" situation. Still today I listen for that special voice to lead me, guide, and direct me.

The next product that Holy Spirit gave me was HotComb-N-Bottle, this was my premier product for a long time. Not trying to reinvent the wheel- but HotComb-N-Bottle was created because of two little girls who were running late for an invent that they were scheduled to participate in. Hear the rest of the story at a seminar coming near you!

N***ow 13 products and eight years later, I have Rxestoratives Hair and Skin Product line to assist hair salons and individuals with their hair.***

The Purpose of this Manual

This guide was created for information purposes only. It is a guide to assist you in understanding your hair and skin better from a natural, holistic or herbal perspective. It can be used during one of our consultation or at a one of Rxestoratives Hair & Skin Seminars. It can certainly be used independently. This guide explains hair dilemmas products, nutrition, vitamins, ingredients and the benefits of them all. This book was designed to be a tool for reference purposes. If you'd like to schedule a live seminar in your local area, please contact us at www.rxestoratives.com or respond to us directly via email at rxestoratives@gmail.com.

Taking care of your hair should not be a hassle it should be easy or simple as washing and conditioning your hair. Stop by any beauty supply store, and you will be immediately overwhelmed, especially if you are not clear as to what you need or why you need it. With our process of cleansing the hair it is simple after you have read this manual shopping for hair and skin products should be a breeze. Once you understand your "Type Hair" it's easy to fine the proper product for you.

This next section is designed to be a place for you to takes notes as you begin your own holistic journey into personal hair care. We've provided lined pages in the back of the guide for you to take notes or make a list to revisit a page. List realizations you find with your own hair.

CHAPTER 2

Let's Get Started!

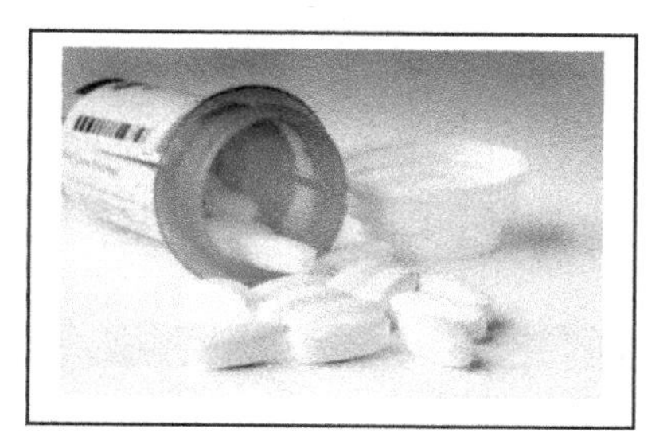

Please take mental notes or use the pages provided in the rear of the book for cross references. I'm sure questions you might have may be found in the pages of this manual or wait for one of RXestoratives Hair & Skin seminars to address your question. We are open for invites.☺

Often, we do not consider the effects that medications have on our hair and skin. Numerous medications have countless side effects that pose potential threats to our hair and skin. Ruminate carefully as you continue your hair journey.

RXestoratives offer one on one consultations. During a one on one consultation, a review of your medication can possibly determine what if any side effects may or may not contributing to hair loss, thinning, dryness, dandruff, and other hair and skin conditions.

Hair Growth Cycles

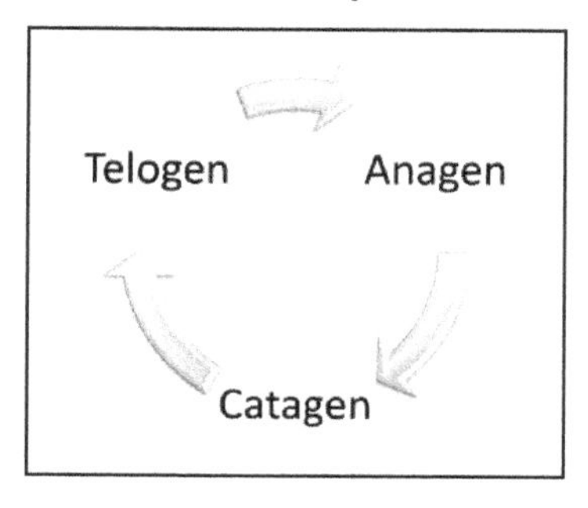

The cycle of hair growth goes through three identified stages – **Anagen** (growing phase) **Telogen** (resting phase), **Catagen** (transitional phase) then back to the **Anagen Phase**. Approximately 90% of hairs are going thru the Anagen phase, then 5% to 10% enter the Telogen phase and ends up in the Catagen phase. In the scalp, the Anagen growth phase lasts between 2 to 6 years, catagen between 2 to 3 weeks, and Telogen between 2 to 3 months. If there are any medical or trauma, or vitamin deficiencies or extreme diet attempt this will disrupt one or more of the Hair Growth Cycles and it greatly affect the hair growing cycles, that ultimately leads to hair loss.

Texture Defined

What is good hair bad hair what kind of hair do you have?
Let's see:

Normal Hair

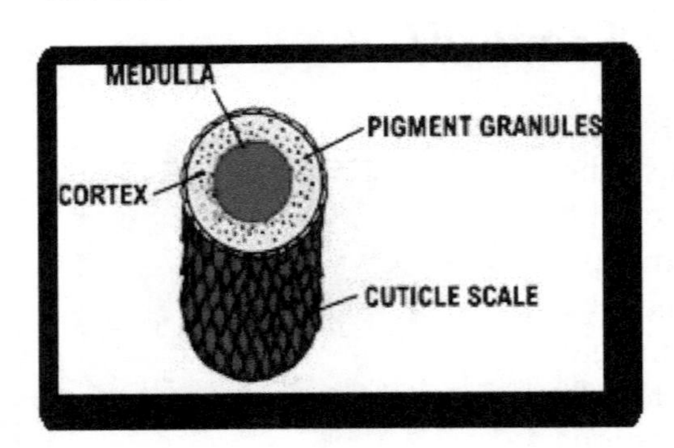

Straight, wavy and curly hair are all examples of "Normal" hair. Healthy hair will have outer cuticles made from dead, keratinized cuticle cells that overlap each other in a fish scale like effect. The outer cuticle is the strongest part of the hair fiber and protects the inner cortex. The inner cortex of the fiber is also made from dead keratinized cells that have been flattened and squeezed together. The difference between straight, wavy, and curly hair is in the shape.

- ❖ Straight hair is circular, or nearly circular in the cross section. In straight hair because of its strength the cross section is circular. (Caucasian) In any direction that the hair grows it receives its direction from a diagonal direction growing across the hair fiber.

- ❖ Wavy hair has a more oval shape to it.

- ❖ Curly hair has a very flat oval shape to it. (African) – In wavy hair the hair fibers overlap and they are oval these hair fibers are stronger but less flexible. The curls will run in the same direction when they are all aligned together and run the same way. It's like a slinky.

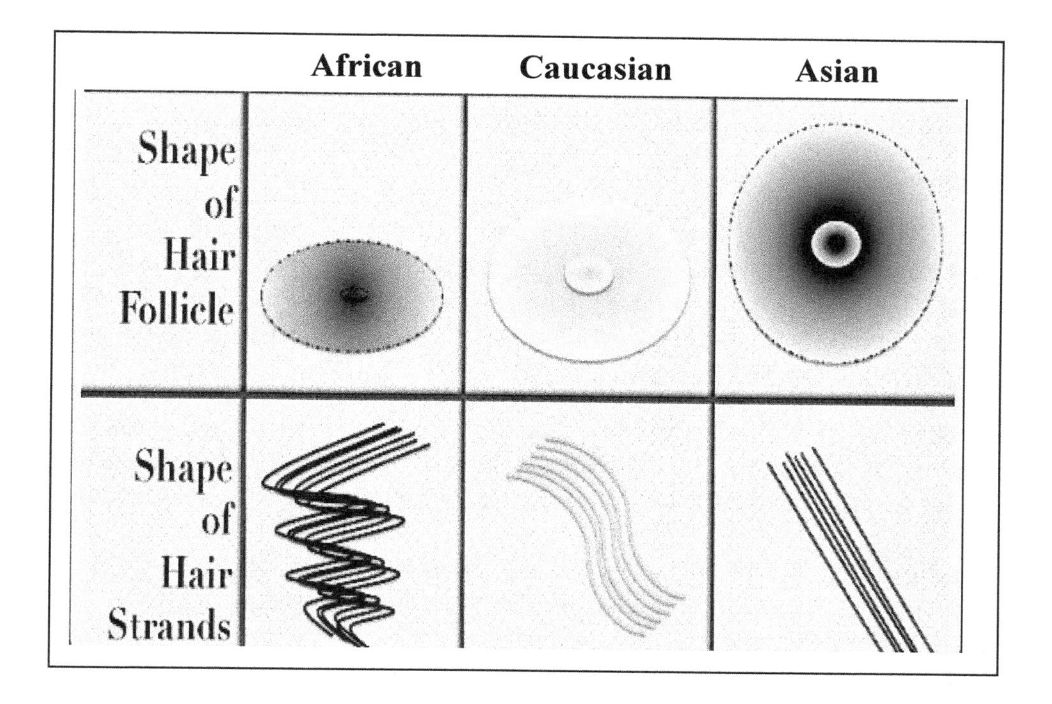

Not surprisingly, curly hair is made by curly hair follicles and straight hair by straight hair follicles. The curl of curly follicles means that when the cells of the hair fiber are incorporated, those that are on the inner curve are flattened less than those on the outer curve. The result is to fix a curl into the hair fiber across the oval cross section. The curl is permanent, and if the hair fiber is pulled and let go, the fiber will spring back into its original curl just as tensile steel springs. Therefore, one side seems to curl better than the other side.

Hair is hair you have hair then you have ***"Normal" hair.***

Types of Hair

To take proper care of your hair it is wise to be educated on the Texture and Type of your hair. Like finger prints and snowflakes no two textures, curls or coils are alike. There are several Hair Typing Systems in place and it is no sense in reinventing the wheel. You have the Andre` Walker System and the L.O.I.S. hair typing system that goes into detail helping us to understand "our hair". We will examine the Andre` Walker Hair Typing System.

There is a lot involved in knowing your Hair type. Knowing the correct curl pattern allow you to choose the best products for your hair. Listed below and in the next few pages let learn about your hair

Texture:

The texture of hair is based on the size or circumference of the hair strand. Cosmetologists classify the texture as being coarse, medium or fine. The texture of hair varies from person to person it even depends on ethnicity or when they are blended: When Caucasian and African ethnicities have children, this is a blend.

- **Coarse** hair has the largest size circumference, and is stronger mainly because it is thicker. This hair/tress is known to be harder to work with as far as chemical processes i.e. relaxer (perms), color, Jheri curl type services.
- **Medium** texture demonstrates the mid-range size of the hair shaft, this hair illustrates very little problems when it comes to styling the hair.
- **Fine** hair is the smallest in circumference shape and is very easy to deal with at ties you do have to monitor chemical services as this hair is easier to become damaged or over processed.

COARSE	The strands in coarse hair are very wide in circumference, making them the strongest of all hair textures. As a result, it's easy to maintain length with coarse hair since it's more resistant to damage.
MEDIUM	Hair with medium width consists of strands that are strong and elastic, and neither too thin nor too thick. Medium width hair is also somewhat resistant to damage, making it easy to maintain length.
FINE	Hair with fine width has a very small circumference and is very delicate and easy to damage. Thus, it's often difficult to maintain length with fine hair. **Deep conditioning** after you wash is a good way to nourish and strengthen fine hair. You'll also want to keep manipulation of your hair to a minimum to avoid unnecessary breakage by reducing your use of combs and brushes and steering clear of elaborate, high-maintenance hairstyles. (Naturally Curlly, 2014)

The parts that make up Hair are Porosity, Density, Width, Length and Type:

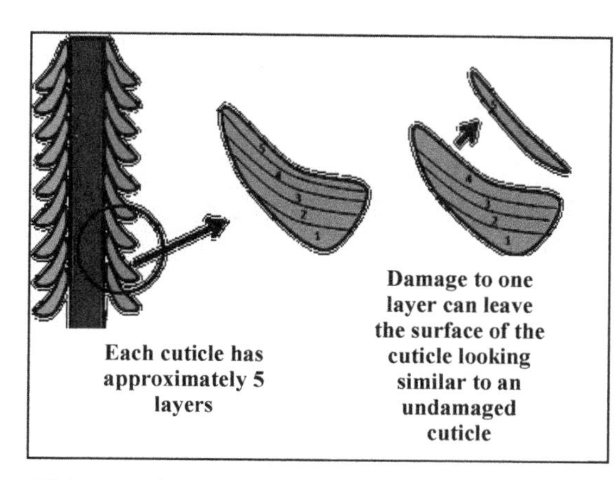

Porosity:

The cuticle has about seven layers of dead keratin on it, and these cuticles overlap each other to make up a strand of hair. Porosity can happen for several reasons. Porosity is damage to the hair strands. It is when holes, breakage or cracks within the strand of hair…. This is when the cuticle has been lifted, leaving chemical processes and hair products…….. For healthy shiny hair, you must know your hair porosity.

There two are quick simple tests you can perform at home to tell your hair's porosity: High, Medium or Low.

- ❖ Use a few strands of your hair and put them into a bowl of water. Allow them to sit in the water for 4 minutes. If your hair is floating, this is an example of low porosity. If the strands of hair sink to the bottom of the bowl, this is an example of high porosity.

- ❖ The next test: With one or two strands of hair, do not pull these strands out. From the tip of the strand, gently slide your fingers to the base of the scalp, while sliding your fingers, feel the strand. if the strands are not smooth but bumpy, this demonstrates the cuticles are open and this is a sign of high porosity. If the finger glides smoothly along the hair, then this is low porosity. If the hair can absorb moisture and oil, then the hair is healthy.

Now that the test is done, how many levels of porosity are there? There are three (3) levels of porosity as mentioned earlier- high, medium and low levels.

Density: is the number of individual hair strands per square inch on the scalp. It is often referred to as being thin, medium, and thick hair. Depending on the density of hair determines how much product you will use. A normal amount of strand is thought to be around 2,000 -2,500 per square inch and over 100,000 per head. Just think God knows every strand of hair on our head. *Matthew 10:30 And even the very hairs of your head are all numbered. Amazing! just a thought…… Selah*

When dealing with the density of the hair one must consider styling the hair. Hair density that is thick will do better with layers as a haircut, for thin hair a blunt hair cut is best. For more volume in people with thin hair, a roller set is best to create an illusion of fuller thicker hair.

Width: Hair width (sometimes called texture) refers to the thickness of *individual strands* of your hair, rather than how much hair you have on your head. Knowing your hair width, along with your unique curl pattern, is very important since it can affect your ability to retain length. to find your hair width, take piece of your hair from a brush or comb and hold it up to the light. If the hair is very wide and easily visible, then you have coarse hair. If it's so thin that you can hardly see it, you have fine hair. If your hair appears neither thin nor coarse, you have medium width hair.[1]

[1] http://www.naturallycurly.com/texture-typing/hair-width

Hair Lengths

In addition to your curl pattern, the length of your hair can determine which products you should use as well as how to apply them. Here are some basic hair care tips and product recommendations based on your hair length.[2]

CHOPPED	**FRESHLY CHOPPED: ½" OR LESS (TWAs)** Requires zero to no maintenance! Keep hydrated with a **daily moisturizer** and a **leave-in conditioner** spray
SHORT	**SHORT: ½" - 2" (TWAs & pixie cuts)** Detangle with fingers Use fingers to apply products If hair is very short, use palm of the hand to rub in circles to create texture For slightly longer hair, twist around finger to create curls and coils
MEDIUM	**MEDIUM: 2" - 10" (shoulder to bra strap length)** Detangle with fingers and follow with a wide tooth comb Use **duckbill clips** to separate hair into sections Apply product from root to tip Tip head upside down and use a diffuser to dry Preserve curls and coils overnight by using a multiple-scrunchie **pineapple method** Use a quarter sized amount of styling product per section
LONG	**LONG: 10"+ (armpit to waist length)** Detangle in sections, first with fingers and following with a wide tooth comb Use **duckbill clips** to separate hair into sections Apply product from root to tip, distributing with fingers Tip head upside down and dry with a hair diffuser, or use the **pixie curl method** Use a scrunchie to **pineapple hair** overnight Use two quarter sized dollops of styling product per section

[2] http://www.naturallycurly.com/texture-typing/hair-length

Hair Types

- **Curl Pattern**: is based on how much wave, coil or curl are in the tresses (hair). It has been put into three categories: Wavy Type 2, Curly Type 3 and Coily Type 4. Below is a chart that defines hair types:

Andre Walker's Curl Typing System

Possibly the most popular system and mainly used by curly girls is the Andre Walker system. Many systems are based on this one. In 1997 he took the standard hairdresser texture classes and expanded it into curl typing. He classified hair into four main categories: Straight – Type 1, Wavy – Type 2, Curly – Type 3 and Kinky – Type 4. Andre created and defined subcategories - a, b, c – within the texture classes.

Type 1- Type 1 is straight hair and is further subcategorized:

- Type 1a – Straight (Fine/Thin) – Hair tends to be very soft, shiny and difficult to hold a curl. Hair also tends to be oily, and difficult to damage.
- Type 1b – Straight (Medium) – Hair has lots of volume & body.
- Type 1c – Straight (Coarse) – Hair is normally bone straight and difficult to curl. Asian women usually fall into this category.

Type 2-Type 2 is wavy and tends to be coarse, with a definite S pattern to it. There are three Type 2 subtypes defined below.

- Type 2a – Wavy (Fine/Thin) – Hair has a definite "S" pattern. Normally can accomplish various styles.
- Type 2b – Wavy (Medium) – Hair tends to be frizzy, and a little resistant to styling.
- Type 2c – Wavy (Coarse) – Hair is also resistant to styling and normally very frizzy; tends to have thicker waves.

Type 3-When this type of hair is wet, it appears to be straight. As it dries, the hair goes back to its curly state. When curly hair is wet it usually straightens out. As it dries, it absorbs the water and contracts to its curliest state. Humidity tends to make this type of curly hair even curlier, or frizzier. Type 3 hair has a lot of body and is easily styled in its natural state, or it can be easily straightened with a blow dryer into a smoother style. Healthy Type 3 hair is shiny, with soft, smooth curls and strong elasticity. The curls are well defined and springy.

Andre Walker[3] defines two subtypes of curly hair. First, there is type 3a and 3b. The longer the hair is the more defined the curl. Then there is type 3b hair, which has a medium amount of curl to tight corkscrews. It's not unusual to see a mixture of these types existing on the same head. Curly hair usually consists of a combination of textures, with the crown being the curliest part. Lastly there is a type 3c. This is a hair type that is not in Andre Walker's book. This type of hair can be described as tight curls in corkscrews. The curls can be either kinky, or very tightly curled, with a lot of strands densely packed together.

- *Type 3a* – Curly (Loose Curls) – Hair tends to be shiny and there can be a combination of textures. It can be thick & full with lots of body, with a definite "S" pattern. It also tends to be frizzy. The longer the hair the more defined the curl becomes.
- *Type 3b* – Curly (Tight Curls) – Also tends to have a combination texture, with a medium amount of curl.

Type 4- According to Andre Walker, if your hair falls into the Type 4 category, then it is kinky, or very tightly curled. Generally, Type 4 hair is very wiry, very tightly coiled and very fragile. Like Type 3 hair, Type 4 hair appears to be coarse, but it is quite fine, with lots and lots of these strands densely packed together. Healthy Type 4 hair typically has sheen rather than shine. It will be soft and silky to the touch and have proper elasticity.

There are two subtypes of Type 4 hair: Type 4a, tightly coiled hair that, when stretched, has an S pattern, much like curly hair; and Type 4b, which has a Z pattern, less of a defined curl pattern. The hair bends in sharp angles like the letter Z. Type 4a tends to have more moisture than Type 4b which will be wiry.

- Type 4a – kinky (Soft) – Hair tends to be very fragile, tightly

[3] https://www.andrewalkerhair.com/

coiled, and has a more defined curly pattern.

- Type 4b – kinky (Wiry) – Also very fragile and tightly coiled; however, with a less defined curly pattern -has more of a "Z" pattern shape.

This information is provided courtesy of NaturallyCurly.com®

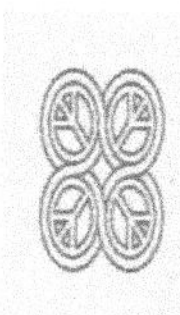

ANDRE WALKER

HAIR TYPING SYSTEM

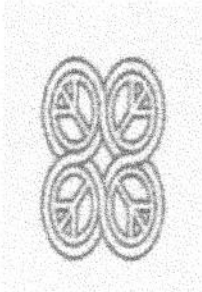

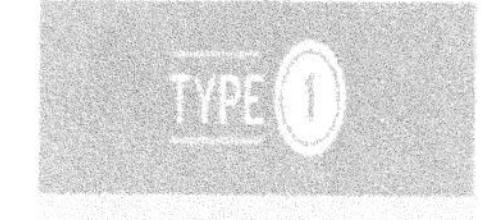

STRAIGHT HAIR

FINE & FRAGILE TO COARSE & THIN (CURL RESISTANT)

TYPE 1 PRODUCTS

- ULTIMATE MOISTURE SHAMPOO
- TKO CONDITIONER
- GET IT STRAIGHT
- O-OIL

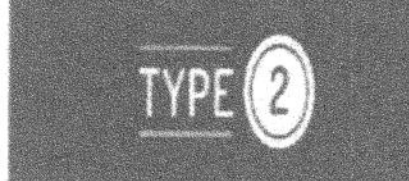

WAVY HAIR

FINE & THIN TO COARSE & FRIZZY

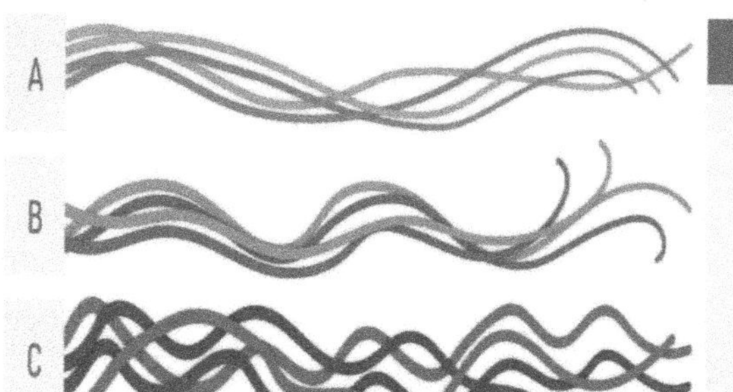

TYPE 2 PRODUCTS

- ULTIMATE MOISTURE SHAMPOO
- TKO CONDITIONER
- BEAUTIFUL CURLS
- GET IT STRAIGHT
- O-OIL

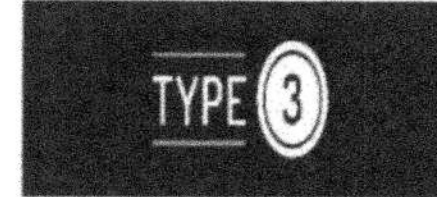

CURLY HAIR

LOOSE CURLS TO CORKSCREW CURLS

TYPE 3 PRODUCTS

- ULTIMATE MOISTURE SHAMPOO
- TKO CONDITIONER
- 3A: BEAUTIFUL CURLS
- 3B: BEAUTIFUL KINKS
- GET IT STRAIGHT
- O-OIL

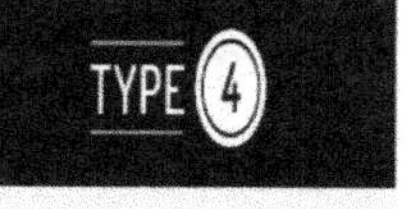

KINKY HAIR

TIGHT COILS TO Z-ANGLED COILS

TYPE 4 PRODUCTS

- ULTIMATE MOISTURE SHAMPOO
- TKO CONDITIONER
- BEAUTIFUL KINKS
- GET IT STRAIGHT
- O-OIL

COILY	CURVY	WAVY

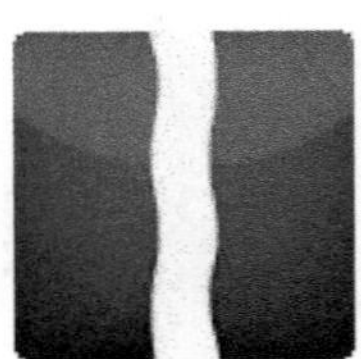

Type 2 - Wavy Hair

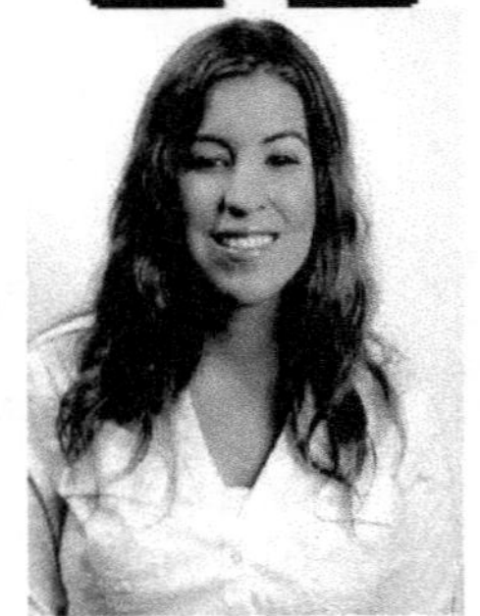

This Type 2 wavy hair pattern has an "S" shape formation when the hair is cut close to the scalp. When the hair grows out or long hair will not bounce up. This is wavy hair not curly. This type hair even when layered will not curl up.

This hair is slightly straight and has a slight curl. This hair tends to be fine in density. It has very little natural sheen and will not have volume or delineation.

This Type 2A hair has more of an elongated "S" waved shape to it. This hair sticks closer to the head. Again, the hair texture is thin and fine in density. This texture does have a slight sheen to it naturally, but still has no volume.

QUICK TIPS

- Use a sealant (*sealant is oil mix with a silicone or just silicone used by itself)* use a lightweight oil: Grapeseed, coconut oil are light weight oils.
- Using a light weight holding spray or spritz is useful: be mindful of the product build up
- Use a low pH 4-6 sulfate free cleanser(shampoo) to achieve body for this 2A type hair.

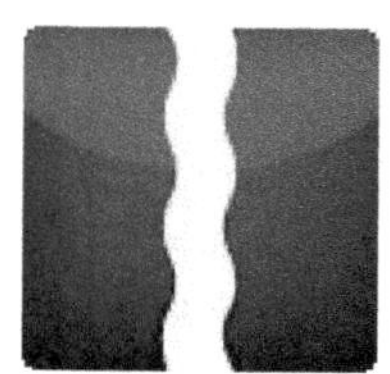

Type 2B - Wavy Hair

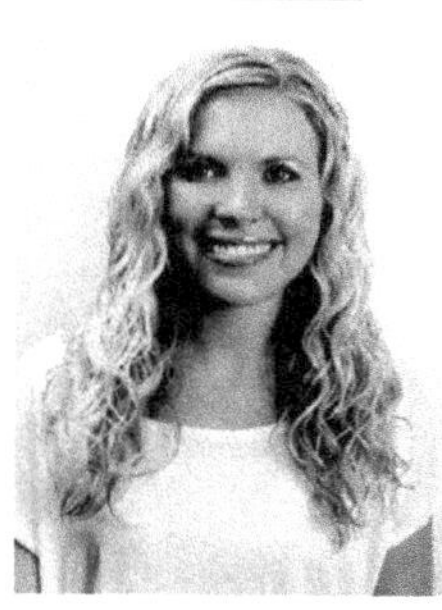

Like in Type 2A hair this type 2B hair has a "S" like wave pattern throughout the hair but loses curl delineation very rapid. The hair is closer to the scalp like 2A but tends to have more frizz than Type 2A. This type seems to be oilier than other hair types.

QUICK TIPS

- Use citrus based products, cleansers, conditioners, leave-in treatments.
- Find products that is two-products in one, moisturizer (light oil based, silicone) and frizz control properties.
- You may use a product that offers light hold.
- To lock your natural, sheen a honey based product is beneficial.
- Try a product that removed oil from your scalp and add volume to the roots of the hair. For more volume.
- Chose a protein treatment based on the hair type and issue (just make sure to choose the Right Protein Treatment page 169.

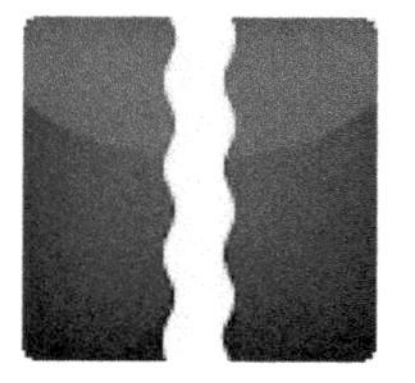

Type 2C - Wavy Hair

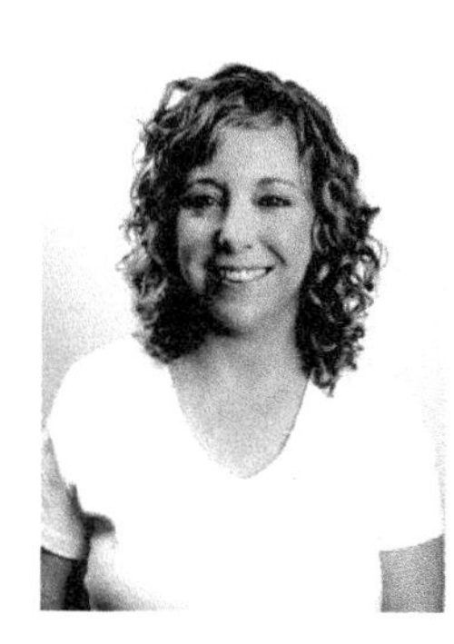

In one Type of hair a style is perfect but with this Type 2C there are very coarse waves and the hair pattern is curly without waves. When using styles like rollers, twist, bantu knots and other similar hair styles; hair loss can occur with wavy hair.

QUICK TIPS

- With this hair, a diffuser was made for this hair.
- Blow dry the hair upside down for full volume, towel dry the hair.

- When applying leave-in product to Type 2C hair apply to hands first almost like lotion then apply to hair, the curls in this type can be scrunched in.
- Use products that accentuate the curls
- Not a lot of oil should be used with Type 2C but will be more affective if used as a Hot Oil treatment, about 3-4 times a year followed with citrus based products (**c**onditioner, **c**leanser, **c**onditioner the RXHSW® way 3C's)

Next Type 3 hair is curly hair, this type hair range from light curls to ringlet curls there are three definition of Type 3 hair. These curls have clear curl definition they offer lots of body naturally, and easy to manage. This hair is not coarse and rarely dry it has a natural shine to it.

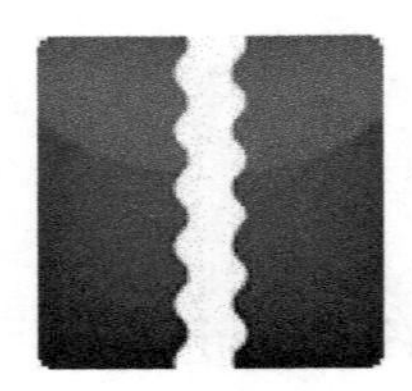

Type 3A - Curly Twirly

First type of 3A is very curly, curl definition is clearly definite. 3A hair is coily and springy very easy to manage and straightened when necessary. Curly hair love hair products even with a natural shine.

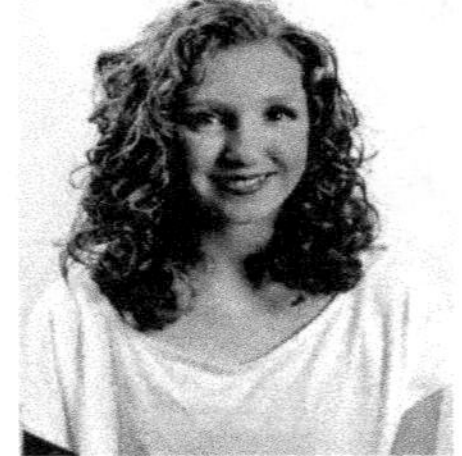

QUICK *TIPS*

- Using moisturizing sulfate free cleanser and a low pH conditioner to achieve the best curl definition for this Type 3A.
- Leave-In conditioner will affectively hydrate and moisturize your curls.
- To keep hair from becoming frizzy use products that are silicone based and find gels and creams that offer light moisturize and great curl delineation.

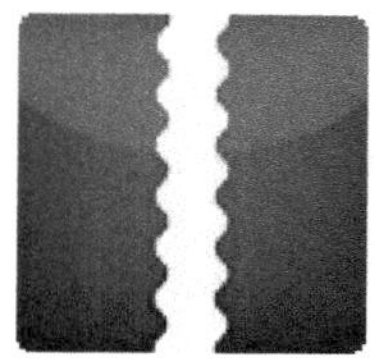

3B - Curly Spirally

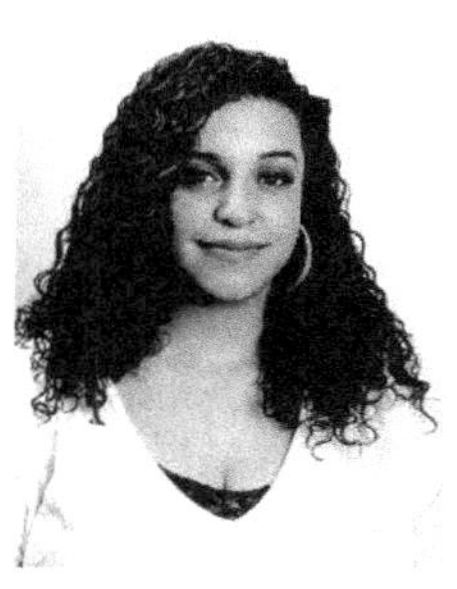

3B Type offers the most ringlet type curls. These curls are bouncy with high definition curly curls. 3B hair tends to be quite coarse compared to the other Types of hair, at times can be difficult to manage and hard to style. With the proper tools and products, the hair can be straightened. A lot of work needs to be done to this type of hair. To reduce the frizz use creams and/or thick gel to set curls.

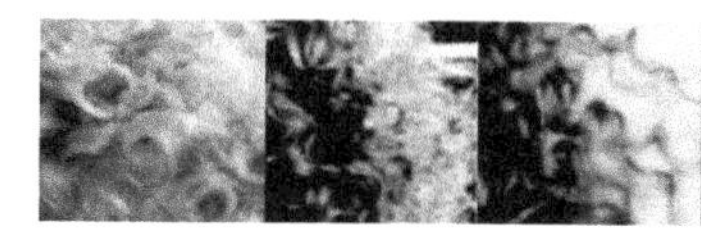
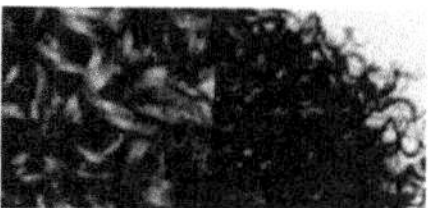

QUICK TIPS

- 3B Hair needs a creamy type cleanser not a clear one this is best for curly springy type hair
- Find a hydrating leave-In Conditioner. My suggestion is ACV30 Leave-in Conditioner by Rxestoratives Hair & Skin Wellness
- Silicone based products works best for frizz control. May I suggest RXHSW® The Glossifier

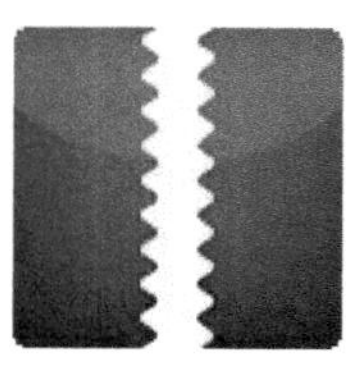

3C - Curly Coily

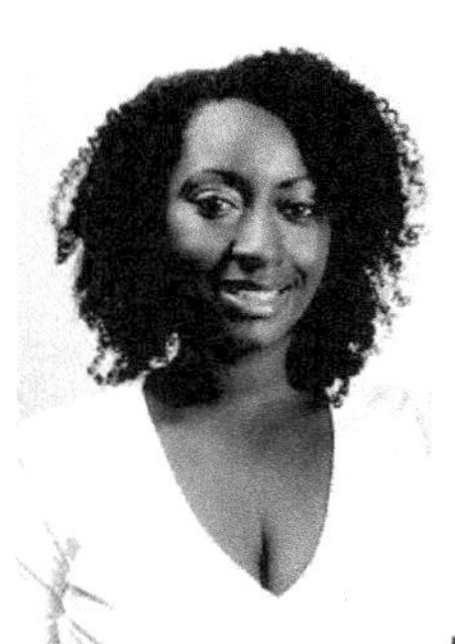

Tight, Coarse corkscrew type 3C hair has very capacious tightly coiled hair. The curls are the size of pencil. The curls may be kinky dull and dry type curls. This hair has a lot of hair in a very small area the hair is densely packed together. Mostly found in African Americans. Styling washing even maintaining this hair type is very challenging. Although there will be a lot of hair the hair itself is fine/thin in texture.

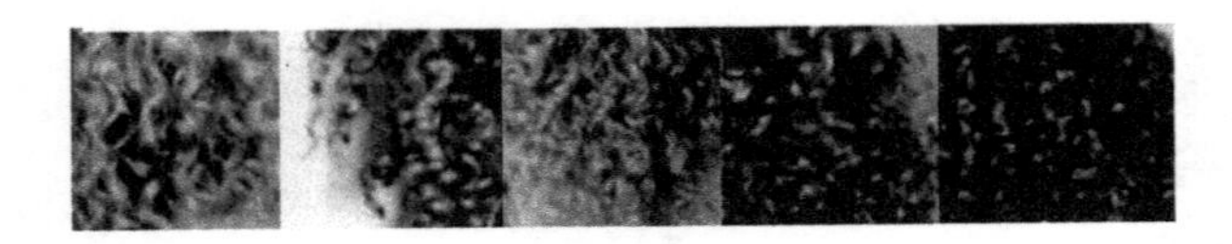

QUICK TIPS

- Moisture is key when dealing with this hair type. Using a cream base shampoo is beneficial. Follow with a thick non-alcohol base conditioner.
- The benefit of oil, natural butters are great to use for moisturizing purposes. Using the RXHSW® 3C's (Conditioner, Cleanser, Conditioner) process you will have great moisturized hair and leaves the hair easy to manage.

Type 4 - Coily Hair

Type 4 hair unlike Type 3 is very deceiving type hair You would think that this hair was like rope however, this hair is very fragile. Coiled hair can range from fine, kinky, thin to wiry thick or coarse strands. The hair consists of many strands which, are densely and closely packed together with tight coiled/curly strands. There are two types of Type 4 hair. This hair does not shine without applying the right products.

As mentioned above, this hair is fragile because Type 4 hair has fewer cuticles per strand unlike the other "Types" of hair. When we decide to put chemicals in this hair type, another layer of cuticles and have less protection from being damaged and become extremely porous affording the hair to hold moisture. it becomes dry brittle and there is breakage.

This fourth type hair tends to rely heavily on chemical relaxers (what we call perms) to manage their hair. Type 4 hair tends not to grow very long unless it's in the 'genes. There are two types of Type 4 Hair textures, Coily Cotton and Coily Coarse.

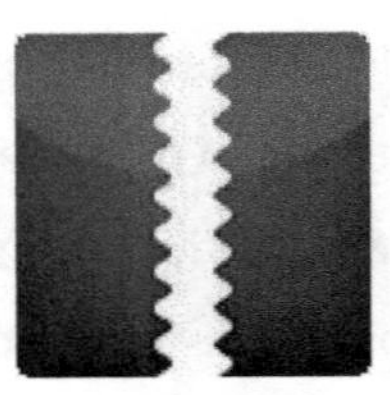

4A - Coily Cotton

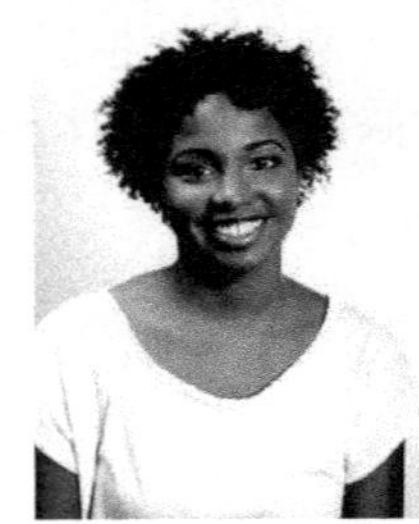

The first is Type 4A unlike 4B has very tight coils and miniature ringlets like the size of a straw (that's why we do "straw sets" at times), it also has an "S" pattern to it. There is more moisture in Type 4A hair than 4B; when right

products are used, you will see a definite curl pattern.
This hair appears to have a lot of hair but it doesn't. The deception comes from there are more strands in one area or all over than in other hair types. This hair shrinkage rate is at a whopping 75%.

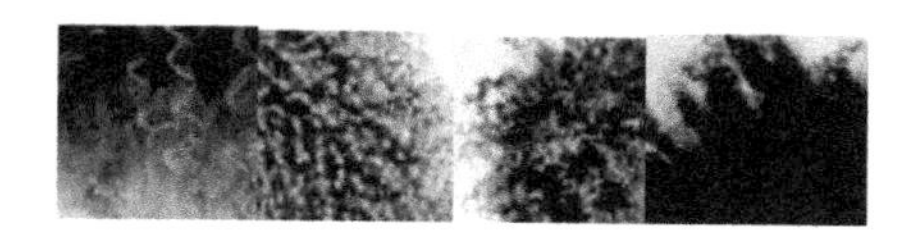

QUICK TIPS

- Try the suggested RXHSW® "3C's" Cleanser process: Conditioner, Cleanser, Conditioner.
- Perform a Baking Soda Treatment at least four times a year: (see treatments in the back of the manual).
- Do not use excessive heat.
- For hair growth follow guide for Essential Oils, choose the best oils for your needs.
- Wrap your hair at night.
- Get professional services done by a professional not a "kitchen beautician."

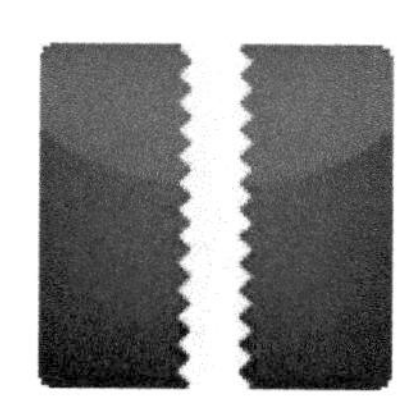

4B - Coily Coarse

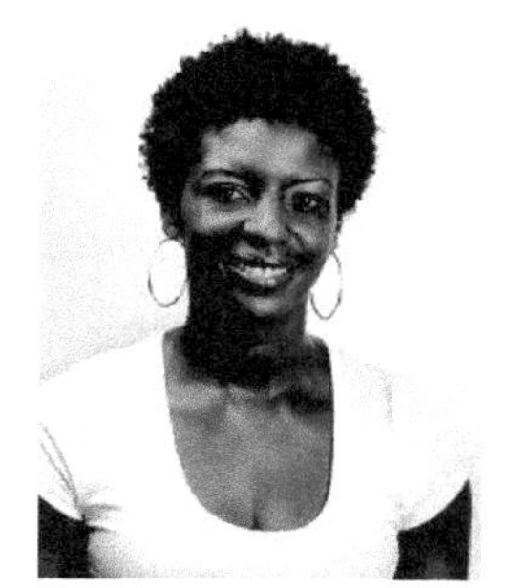

This second type 4B texture is hard to hold curls without chemical or heat.

4B: Has a kinky wiry "Z" pattern, less defined curl pattern, this hair type hair "Z" shape (like stairs) patterns in the hair. It's more of a cotton kinky like texture. The wave pattern comes in various size and patterns. The actual length of this hair is only seen when straightened out. Again, as with this hair the shrinkage rate is phenomenal. Most of Type 4A applies to 4B its just more of a cotton type of tresses (hair).

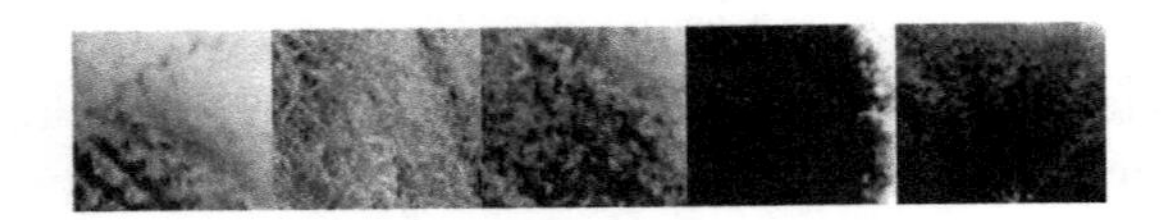

QUICK *TIPS*

- Find the best carrier oils for your texture, highly moisturizing oil: Coconut Oil, Grapeseed Oil.
- Try the suggested RXHSW® Cleanser process: Conditioner, Cleanser, conditioner.
- Perform a Baking Soda Treatment at least four times a year: (see treatments in the back of the manual).
- Do not use excessive heat.
- For hair growth follow guide for Essential Oils, choose the best oils for your needs.
- Wrap your hair at night.
- If the hair is natural plat the hair down to air dry it and to protect it, old wife's tales use a satin cap or pillow case.
- Get professional services done by a professional not a "kitchen beautician" ☺

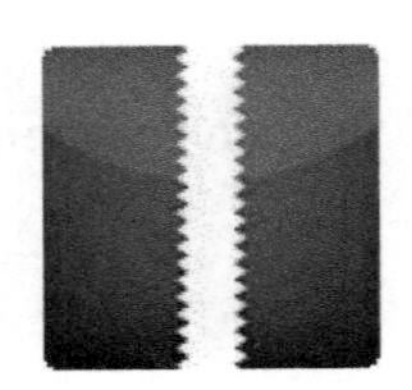

4C - *Coily Ziggly*

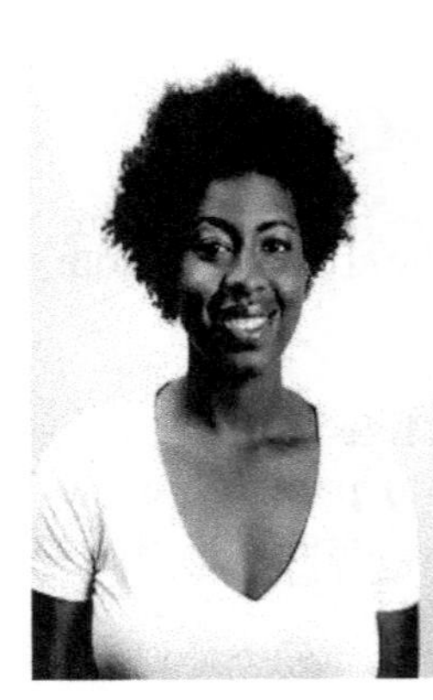

Type 4C like the others mentioned earlier is a very challenging type of hair. There is really no curl or wave formation no "Z" shape coils, no real curl definition. This Type hair does not retain water, making this hair susceptible to dryness and breakage quicker than the other hair Types. This is due to how the hair grows, the cuticles are very tight and closed making it hard to receive moisture or to retain it as well.

It comes in fine thin and coarse hair. It can be soft, rough wiry, dry or dull to the touch. It resembles the other Type 4 hair and the shrinkage rate is at almost 100x's it length.

QUICK TIPS

- Find the best carrier oils for your texture, highly moisturizing oil: Basix® (sold by Rxestoratives Hair & Skin Wellness), Silicone base oil.
- Do the suggested RXHSW® Cleanser process: Conditioner, Cleanser, Conditioner.
- Perform a Baking Soda Treatment at least eight times a year: (see treatments in the back of the manual).
- Hot Oil Treatments should be done first if the hair is damaged then the RXHSW® Cleanser process, or performed at least 12-18 times a year as well.
- Use wide tooth combs for this Type of hair.
- If you or your daughter have a massive amount of hair, you might consider putting 6-8 twist, braids in the hair to treat the hair. Yes, part the hair into 6-8 sections do light braids or twist rinse the hair, apply the product following the RXHSW® Cleanser process rinse well when finish undo the hair and with a wide tooth comb, comb out the hair and dry as usual its best to repeat the first step and either air dry or place under the hooded dryer for 15 minutes no more than 25 minutes to style as usual.
- If you choose to wear your hair natural, find a thick creamy hair pudding to help make the hair longer.
- Do not use excessive heat.
- For hair growth follow guide for Essential Oils, choose the best oils for your needs.
- Wrap your hair at night.
- If the hair is natural plat the hair down to air dry it and to protect it, old wives' tales use a satin cap or pillow case.
- Get professional services done by a professional not a "kitchen beautician". ☺

These statements have not been evaluated by the Food and Drug Administration. This product is not intended to diagnose, treat, cure, or prevent any disease.

For your hair health: Protein-rich Diet

For hair, skin and nails a very important part of growth is producing keratin. A diet high in protein helps the body to create keratin. To fight against hair loss, and to encourage new healthy hair growth, add foods rich in protein such as dairy: eggs, dairy, yogurt, soy, poultry, fish, lean beef, and nuts to your weekly shopping list. Again, what goes in is what comes out what comes out.

Finding the Right Products for Your Type Hair

Fine Hair

African fine thin hair is vastly different from Caucasian fine thin hair. Caucasian hair tends to be oilier, and African hair tends to be more dull and dry. To keep your hair as healthy and happy as possible, you need to know what type of conditioner to treat it with **Use volumizing conditioner on fine, flat hair.**[1] If you have straight, silky hair with no frizzing problems, you want a conditioner that's going to add some much-needed texture to hair that might otherwise seem to just hang from your head. Volumizing conditioner is lighter than a regular conditioner, and doesn't add extra weight to hair when used regularly.

People with fine, flat hair should never use smoothing conditioners; these heavy products will make your hair lifeless, very flat, and oily.

Look for a light weight moisturizing conditioner if you have wavy hair. Wavy hair can be hard to work with — in humid weather it can frizz out of control, and in dry weather it can grow limp. The more curl there is in a strand of hair, the dryer the end of the strand gets, because it's hard for the natural oils from the scalp to wind their way down a curled strand than a straight one. Although wavy hair doesn't tend to be as dry as curly hair, you still need a moisturizing conditioner to stand in for those oils that aren't making their way down to the tips of your hair.

- Wavy hair can be flattened out either by humid weather, or conditioners that are "moisturizers" that is too heavy on the hair.

Find products that are specifically for wavy hair.

Curly Thick Hair

Thick Curly hair has to be moisturized with a deep-hydrating conditioner.[2] Fi Find a products that addresses this issue. Very curly hair tends to be very dry. If you have thick, curly hair, odds are that without a deep-hydrating conditioner that is oil based the hair will be dry and become extremely dry and frizzy. Sebum is located at the base of the scalp and will flow down to the ends of the tresses. Look for conditioners labeled as "deep hydrating" or for curly hair specifically.

- You should also consider using a leave-in conditioning mask on a weekly or bi-weekly basis. These conditioners are meant to be left in your hair for 10-15 minutes, then washed out like regular conditioner. With regular use, you should see a significant change in the way your curls hold together rather than frizzing away.

- You should also purchase leave-in conditioner that's oil based in spray form. You can spray this product onto your hair when it's either dry or wet to keep it soft and hydrated. Remember not all oils are oily.

Protect the intense curl in African hair with a deep-hydrating conditioner or oil based products. African hair is known to be defined as "kinky". However, with the right conditioning products, even the curliest hair can be shiny and healthy. When purchasing products for your hair look for hair products that loaded with oils like: Shea butter, Coconut Oil,

Peanut Oil, Castor Oil, Moroccan Argon Oil these are designed to boost moisture in African American hair like no other products can.

Look for products that say: "hydrating," "moisturizing," "balancing," or, if you have wavy or curly hair, "curly."

- SHAMPOO- Although this is unrelated to conditioners, you shouldn't shampoo your hair regularly. Shampoo every 7-10 days — every 14 days at the minimum. NOTE: Look for a shampoo that is creamy
- Over-shampooing will strip the hair of natural oils, causing even more dryness and counteracting the positive benefits of your conditioning routine.
- And by adding a **HOT OIL** treatment for your hair is most beneficial. The formula for Hot Oil treatment is in Chapter 14.

Find a conditioner that is color safe or a color-depositing conditioner.

As time passes after the initial color application, you'll notice that the color/dye in your hair will get begin to fade or look washed out. To keep the color vibrant for as long as you possibly can, you'll want to choose the appropriate color conditioner (conditioner for hair with color).

- Using hair products (shampoo, conditioner, gel sprays) contributes to this process. When possible, find a color rinse to add to the shampoo, and conditioner to keep your color vibrant longer. If you consider yourself an advance kitchen beautician, (do this at your discretion) find your color a DEMI color (No PERMANENT COLOR AT ALL – Zero)! Mix 1oz of your matching Demi color to 1oz of 10 volume (add 1 tablespoon (T) of water, 1 teaspoon (tsp) of oil), mix well. Add to the shampoo, follow the 3 C's procedure and style as usual.

- Color safe conditioners as we know seal hair cuticles, which allows your hair to hold onto the dye for a longer period of time. Look for packaging that advertises it is "sulfate free," "color-safe," "color extend, or that is "color care" type of conditioner.
- Color-depositing conditioners, if you can find the conditioner that complements the color, like the same company of the color, this conditioner will deposit a small amount of color each time it's applied to the hair. So, this will not only maintain the richness of the original color, but also cover the roots that emerge as your hair grows out for a period of time.
- Make sure to choose a shade of color-depositing conditioner that matches your dyed color.

CHAPTER 3

Hair Loss Prevention (Dietary)

A diet with iron, silica and calcium help to reduce even prevent hair loss. Vegetable high in minerals are green leafy vegetables when they are not over cooked. Eating any type of oats raw are full of silica plus dried dehydrated fruits even cherry juice are high in iron.

For women, hair loss or thinning could be a sign for ailments and deficiencies in the body, such as problems with the gastrointestinal tract. This would be a signal of inadequate acids in the stomach; or it could be a sign of low protein, zinc and other nutrients beneficial for healthy hair. There are simple home remedies that facilitate healthy hair. Something simple as drinking milk containing acidophilus, also comes in the form of a tablets as well. **Just a suggestion; This is not to diagnose or treat any medical issues. Please see your physician for consultation.**

For men, dealing with the "norm" male pattern baldness, scientists have determined this process can be slowed down by consuming a low-fat diet. With high levels of testosterone men during puberty will experience thinning hair loss at an earlier age. Eating a diet high in protein and not vegetable protein, but a meat derived protein diet and that's high in fat will help lower testosterone levels. It's been noted prior to WWII Japanese, Chinese had less thinning and baldness because their diets are high in meat protein and have less fatty diet. Remember eating healthy foods rich in meat protein based foods won't stop hair loss but may slow down hair loss.

With an increased higher level of testosterone during puberty some scientist suggest that this contributes to early male pattern baldness. With men adhering to a low-fat diet, and the proper supplements this may be reversed or slowed down. With a diet that is high in protein from meat (beef), raises the testosterone levels. Which contribute to balding/thinning via the follicles. These high levels truly affect the hair follicles when there is an abundance of testosterone in the body.

Before World War II, male pattern baldness was indeed rare in Japanese men. They (the males) consumed far less beef than the American males. Their diets were more grains, fruits, vegetables and fish. Whereas the American diet was more processed foods and high in beef. Please Note: Eating low fat foods may not stop hair loss; but it might help slow down the hair loss.

One of the most prevalent causes of hair loss is Anemia. By eating foods rich in iron-rich like liver any organ meat, whole grain cereals, steamed: leafy dark green vegetables like: kale, collards, turnip greens, Swiss chard, broccoli, even cabbage, eggs, raisins, cranberries, dates, may assist in reversing stopping slowing down the process of hair loss. For Women; (Please Note: Avoid if you are pregnant)

The composition of hair is made of mostly protein. With a diet rich in protein this encourages hair growth. A recommended-suggested diet for healthy hair growth would/should include the food mentioned above. Plus, by adding: brewer's yeast, wheat germ, and two tablespoons of granulated lecithin, along with protein from beef not vegetable protein, these foods which are also high in B vitamins as mentioned earlier an important nutrient for hair.

In Europe, there are studies that supports soy protein fortifies hair growth and stimulates hair growth up to 15%. Eating foods that are soy based are an excellent form of obtaining soy protein. Another source of food protein and not meat protein is Low fat cheese (water based cheese) eggs, fish beans lentils, brewer’s yeast and yogurt.

In other countries, there are studies that show the benefits of using Silica. This mineral is very important for having healthy hair, its known to decrease the thinning process. This mineral is found on the outer covering of the potato (when the potato is cut up- that outer covering that turns colors when exposed to oxygen is a form of silica), it's found in green and red peppers and cucumbers as well, these vegetables are high in silica. Another food excellent for obtaining silica is eating bean sprouts or any sprouted foods. When added to shampoo, it is known to prevent baldness and it stimulates hair growth and offers beautiful sheen to the hair (tresses).

Suggested Hair Vitamin &
Supplement Hair Product Regimen

Vitamin/ Supplement	Defined
Liquid Silica	Silica is needed for bones, nails, joints, hair and skin. Liquid form is the best- it enters our system without going thru the digestive system most beneficial for hair, "Silicon helps hair grow thicker and stronger. Hair with higher silicon content tends to fall out less and has more shine and luster.
Horsetail Tea form or Supplement	Horsetail has a high level of silica. Silica as mentioned above. The Herb or tea form of Horsetail is believed to improve blood circulation. With good circulation, it offers healthier hair follicles and will help men and women who are struggling with hair loss.
Vitamin D	Vitamin D has been known to help reduce hair loss. When there is a deficiency in vitamins it prevents the hair follicles from functioning properly. Vitamin D Receptors: (VDRs) contribute to hair follicle growth cycles, anagen (the growing cycle) and telogen (the resting cycle). This vitamin has the ability to stimulate the hair follicle. Vitamin D also activates the cells within the hair shaft. Healthy cells encourage healthier the hair shafts.

Horsetail Usage

300 mg of the extract three times daily is a normal dose for in either forms. Horsetail preparations should be kept away from sunlight, it should be in dark container or jar that is tight secure and sealed.

Using Horsetail in a dried herbal tea form should be as follows:

- ❖ 2 – 3 teaspoonsful of the tea infused in hot water steep for 5 – 10 minutes.
- ❖ Three times a day.

As a liquid horsetail tincture preparations, the ratio is (1:5), and the recommended dosage is

- ❖ 1 – 4 ml (milliliter)
- ❖ 3 times daily

Vitamin D Usage

Anyone 70 years of age and younger should digest 15 micrograms of Vitamin D per day is the or 12-20 ng/ml. People who are borderline deficient with Vitamin D hair thinning will begin and bones will start to deteriorate. The best range of consumption for Vitamin D 20-50 ml per day for optimal health.

Omega 3 Dietary/Usage (from highest to lowest)

- **Fish – Any Saltwater Fish: Herring, Sardines, Mackerel, Salmon, Halibut, Tuna (fresh not can), Cod, Catfish, Flounder, Grouper, Mahi Mahi**
- **Shellfish – Mussels, Clams, Crab, Lobster, Oysters, Shrimp,**
- **Nuts and Seeds – Chia Seeds, Flax seed, Almond, Pumpkin Seeds, Sunflower Seeds and**
- **Oils – Canola oil,**

It is best to consume Omega 3 supplements is by means of, fish oil in liquid or capsules.

Nutritional doctors recommend one tablespoon of fish oil or 1 – 2 capsules of fish oil daily. This will assist in preventing hair loss and will encourage hair regrowth. At these doses, Omega 3 encourages the **Anagen** growth phase of hair follicles and reduces hair loss during the **Telogen** phase. It also reduces skin inflammation and oils dry scalps.

Since Vitamin E is known to be fat-soluble antioxidant, by adding Omega 3 fatty acids to your daily vitamin supplement regimen will help deprivation through oxidation.

Do not exceed the daily recommended dosage. Omega 3 doses in excess i.e.: 4000mg + can increase the risk of bleeding. [4]

Diagnosis for Hair Loss

Type of Haïr Loss : Traction alopecia

Signs: Steady hair loss around the temples or in the stress areas (e.g. where a ponytail is normally positioned where braids/twist were or tracks for weave hairstyles).

Reasons: The most common cause in natural hair loss is tight braiding and tight hair styles.

Treatment: Several months may past before the Traction alopecia becomes noticeable. It is a scarring affect of alopecia which indicates that the use of certain hair styles may put a strain on hair follicles. With these types of hairstyles, the follicles are destroyed and new hair will not grow. There are ways to avoid hair loss from happening. If the follicles and hair is still present but thinning is visible, this is a positive sign that the follicle has not closed, and regrowth is still possible.

Preventative action is always best (i.e. No! tight braiding hair styles which pull hair tightly). Hair transplants are a possible solution for some cases, but try to avoid these hairstyles completely.

[4] www.progressivehealth.com/hair-loss-omega-3.htm

Treatment for Traction Alopecia

If the follicles are still visible, then stimulation is needed for hair growth- find herbs essential oils that are stimulants.

2oz Carrier Oil	4 drops Horsetail
4 drops Burdock Root	4 drops Stinging Nettle
4 drops Peppermint	2 drops of Rosemary

Warm oil to 90°F let cool for ten minutes. Add essential oils to the carrier oil. Pour final product in dark glass bottle dropper or eye drop bottle. Let product sit for 1 (one) week and shake the product daily.

Use on the scalp as needed 3-4 times per week massage product into comprised areas. If you can do so; wash the hair three (3) times a week with our process RXHSW system. On the first day, follow all steps using the second time only conditioner if you purchase our Step 1&3 This is a stimulating conditioner. Follow with our ACV30, or make your version of an apple cider vinegar leave-in-conditioner, style as usual.

Diagnosis for Hair Loss

Type of Hair Loss: **Traction Alopecia**

Signs: Gradual hair loss around the temples or in an area of stress (e.g. where a ponytail is normally secured where braids/twist were or tracks for weave hairstyles)

Reasons: The most common cause in natural hair is tight braiding and tight hair styles.

Quick Tip #2

Horsetail, Coltsfoot and Nettle under a microscope resemble hair. Certain fruit and vegetables strengthen certain parts of the body. *For example*: **Carrots** are round like eyes, **Avocado** the uterus, **Celery** good for bones, **Figs** good for production of male sperm, **Beans** are shaped like the kidneys, **Sweet Potato** the pancreas, **Grapefruit** for breast and is known to have limoniods which ward off cancer. **Olives** shaped like Ovaries, **Tomato** cut open resembles the heart chambers.

Treatment: Traction alopecia can take several months to become noticeable. Scarring form of alopecia means the long-term use of a specific hair style will cause the destroying of hair follicles, therefore new hair will not grow. Preventative measures are possible, if the hair is still present, thinning and may indicate the follicle has not closed.

Preventative action is always best (i.e. avoid tight braiding/hair styles that pull hair tight). Hair transplants are a possible solution for some cases.

Another Type of Hair Loss:
Trichotillomania alopecia- pronounced- **Tri•cho•till•o•man•ia**

Signs: Trichotillomania alopecia is a mental disorder, where a person pulls out and or plucks out their own hair. The person is not aware of this condition which, is diagnosed by a psychologist. Unconsciously, the person may pull and twist the hair out until the scalp is bald. The person may also pull hair from their eye lashes and the eyebrows.

Reasons: The common cause is hair being pulled in the same spot repeatedly.

Treatment: When diagnosed by a doctor, medication is needed and psychiatric help may be necessary. Damaged hair from Trichotillomania can grow back if the follicles are still open.

Reasons for Hair Loss
Other possible reasons for unnecessary hair loss, thinning, or breakage may be due to:

- Damage from or misuse of hair care products, such as relaxers, permanent color, perms and from flat irons, hot rollers, curling irons, or hair dryers.

- Hair-pulling or hair-twisting habits, braiding to tight, ponytails, weave in the hair which is applied with glue.
- Side effects from medicines or medical treatments, such as chemotherapy or radiation therapy.
- Recent surgery, illness that accompanies high fever, or emotional stress. If there has been a lot of hair loss 4 weeks to 3 months after severe physical or emotional stress, then this type of hair loss stops within a few months.
- Certain diseases, such as lupus and hyperthyroidism involves hair loss.
- Heavy metal poisoning, such as thallium or arsenic poisoning will cause hair loss.
- Poor nutrition and lack of protein or iron in the diet leads to thinning and hair loss.
- Possible damage to the hair shafts from cuts burns or other injuries head injuries
- Scalp issues dandruff, prolonged psoriasis and other scalp issues leads to hair loss.

Regimens Guideline for Thinning Hair

Long before the advent of chemical or surgical hair restoration, people around the world used natural remedies to nourish the scalp and keep hair thick and healthy. There are several common causes for hair loss; stress, imbalanced thyroid, skin infection, medications, age, heredity, and sudden change in weight or diet. Whatever your issue may be, the best remedies listed in the chart and the formulas listed in Chapter 12 may assist in restoring, re-growing, or thickening, your hair.

Based on our tests and trials in dealing with Alopecia, dandruff and hair growth, the EOs[5] that stimulate hair growth have been used with great

[5] EOs – Essential Oils

results but have not been certified by the FDA. With the use of herbs used in treatments for over 100 years, there is yet to be a controlled study to evaluate the evidence that these herbs work. Presently, we can only base our findings on our proven facts that the formulas work.

Achieving great-looking healthy hair with EOs and herbs is not difficult, nor should it be expensive. With a few drops of EOs, herbs, and flowers, added to the right carrier oil, you can create a variety of treatments for the quick restoring of the hair.

Listed within this guide are Essential Oils (EO) formulas that are suggested for thinning hair. When creating treatments; DO NOT OVER INDUGLE IN EO. To create a hair treatment or formula, research the best essential oil therapy for your hair. Make small batches until you thoroughly understand **how to make hair/skin treatments**.

CHAPTER 4

Gray Hair

If we could slow the progression in the aging cycle of our hair turning gray, some of us would be interested in the solution. However, for those who live for the day in which our hair will turn gray, following is an explanation about the graying cycle. The gray hair is white and not gray. There is an internal chemical break down which occurs. There is an enzyme in our bodies called catalase, a natural occurring hydrogen peroxide which increases on our hair. There are other enzymes that would prevent this from happening, but apparently is damaged, has stopped doing its job, or decreases. Subsequently, this decrease causes a malfunction in our hair and it begins to turn white.

To keep your gray hair white, try the following whitening treatment:

- ❖ Use a baking soda rinse at least four times a year. Baking soda is beneficial for the scalp and removes product build up.
- ❖ One (1) cup of baking soda, add enough water to make a paste. Use your judgement in making the paste; not watery (a thick paste)
- ❖ Apply to the hair, and refer to the rest of the instructions in the Treatment section of the book.

□ ***Natural Treatments for Gray Hair***

One popular natural treatment for gray hair is blackstrap molasses. Molasses and gray hair treatment seem to work well together because molasses is full of iron, calcium, magnesium, and many more nutrients. There is no harm in taking a few teaspoons of the substance, and it just might take away your gray hair!

Making sure you have plenty of nutrients, especially vitamin B, is crucial to preventing and treating premature gray hair. Specifically, the B vitamins that help the condition are para-aminobenzoic acid, pantothenic acid, and inositol. Eating yogurt every day seems to help the body to produce these vitamins on its own. Another option is to take a B vitamin supplement to help. Calcium is also important in working with gray hair. If gray hair is already present, adding carrots, bananas, fish, and other fresh veggies and fruit to the diet is claimed to have put the color back into gray hair.

Vitamins/Nutrients to Prevent Gray Hair

To prevent gray hair

4 ounces of Dark Amber Bottle
1.5 ounces of Carrier Oil for your type hair
1 ounces (Use another carrier oil for your hair type (dandruff prone, thinning)
5 drops of Rosemary EO.
5 drops of Sage E. O.
15 drops of Burdock Root
5 drops of Licorice

Warm Carrier oil to normal temperature (120°). Add let cool add EOs. Seal bottle and let sit for 24-48 hours then apply to the hair as often as needed.

- □ Graying hair is caused by a lack of an amino acid called phenylalanine, an amino acid that, in combination with enzymes in the hair, turns it into melanin, the pigment that is responsible for coloring the hair. Phenylalanine is found in nuts, all dairy products, meats, eggs, or in capsules.
- The best way to cure gray hair is through prevention, and the best prevention is a healthy diet. Making sure to eat a diet that is rich in fruits and vegetables is the best way to prevent gray hair. Also, eliminating unnecessary stress in your life will help to keep the gray hair at bay. Taking care of your skin and scalp will also decrease your risk of developing premature gray hair.

- Some of the most common causes of gray hair are mental concerns. Hair is comprised of dead skin cells, so the condition of the skin completely affects the condition of the hair. When a person has many worries on their minds, the skin on the scalp becomes extremely tense. When this happens, the hair follicles do not receive the nutrients they need to produce quality hair. As such, the hair becomes unhealthy and turns gray. Other mental problems include fear and anxiety, which rob the hair of needed scalp marrow. Emu oil is loaded with deep penetrating Omega 3's. Emu oil is known as the follicle awakener and has been used by many to help prevent the onset of gray hair. This oil is also loaded with proteins!

- Diet can also harm the color of your hair. Vitamin B is often called the gray hair vitamin, because if you do not get enough of this vitamin in your diet, your hair will turn gray. Getting enough vitamins and other nutrients in your diet is crucial to having healthy hair and scalp condition.

- Adding B vitamin, the gray hair vitamin, to your diet is important to decrease your risk of developing gray hair before your time. If premature gray hair happens to you, take advantage of gray hair natural remedies before you turn to expensive, and sometimes harmful, hair dyes.

Formula to darken gray hair

For those who have gray hair and desire an alternative to chemical color, visit the website: **www.myhairprint.com/products.** Select the information for your hair type.

Formula to darken Gray hair (at home)

Do this on a regular basis to impact your gray hair:

Coffee 1 ½ Cup of coffee grounds (or Black Tea)
Fresh Sage, several leaves or twigs
Rosemary, 1T
Distilled water, 3-4 C.

Boil the water, add the coffee or black tea bags. Remove from stove add Sage Rosemary let all ingredients cool. Strain the herbs first. Have an additional bowl to catch the liquid to reuse and reapply to hair.

Wash Hair the RXHSW way. Then, pour mixture over the hair repeatedly, place a plastic cap on for 45 minutes or more use your judgement no heat is required but may be useful up to 15 minutes, keep the cap on the hair for 45 minutes.

Follow with a rinse and conditioner. Style as usual.

CHAPTER 5

Braids and Weaves

Braids and Weaves offer a versatile ways to wear your hair. The styles include cornrows, French braids, braid extensions, or thick "African" braids. Stylist applying either braids, cornrows, or weave should remember not to pull the hair too tight to prevent hair loss and headaches.

Hair braids have the potential to cause hair loss and slow hair growth especially when braided to tight. It's common to see receding hair lines from hair braids that have been worn for years. Consequently, it is important to keep the hair and scalp clean and healthy, particularly if hair braids are the primary style for your hair.

Braids are usually wound together very tightly. Consider how difficult it must be for the nutrients in shampoos, conditioners, and oils to completely and thoroughly penetrate each hair follicle. It's a common misconception that shampooing once a week is all the nutrition braids or weaved hair needs. Unfortunately, this is not enough for optimum hair health. The best way to insure your hair braids have the right amounts of nutrition is by treating the hair from the inside out. This ensures each hair follicle has the vitamins, minerals, and amino acids it needs to be healthy. Healthy hair requires daily maintenance and nutrition. See the section on **Food for Thought**. Your hair braids can be heathy with proper treatments, eating the suggested foods, and taking appropriate nutrients for healthy hair.

Helpful Tips Dealing with Braids, Weaves Cornrows

- ❖ Wash braided hair once a week with a conditioner followed with a natural hair oil. **This step is very important**.
- ❖ When taking out braids/weave, the night before add a natural oil to the hair, preferably choose a thick consistency oil like Castor Oil or Our own HotCombNBottle, RXHSW® *. Apply generously.
- ❖ At a minimum of 12 to 24 hours after applying the natural oil to the hair, precede to take braids, plats, or weave out.
- ❖ After the hair (weave) is completely out with a wide tooth comb, comb through hair thoroughly before washing or wetting hair, if not this leads to matted & knotted hair.
- ❖ Use the suggested natural method for washing hair the RXHSW® way. Followed with a natural Leave-In Conditioner a vinegar based Leave-in ACV30* sold by RXHSW® * and oil the scalp well. A suggested oil is Oils of Nature sold by RXHSW®. *

NOTE:

If you are in a phase of actively growing out your hair, AFTER CUTTING YOUR HAIR, you may want to supplement your diet with silica. Some nutritional experts also recommend liver, brewer's yeast, wheat germ, and granulated lecithin to help your body process the protein. Visit your local health food store and ask to speak to a counselor who will help you make good choices about diet and the use of supplements. When you are trying to grow hair, vitamins and supplements help.

You may purchase them from Rxestoratives Hair and Scalp Wellness Center or online at www.rxestoratives.com.

During this process, it may take a few months for new hair growth or even up to a year. It totally depends on how fast your hair grows. Supplementing it with the right vitamins may help in this area. Understand with the right system you don’t have to cut off your hair to transition from chemical to natural. The key to growing out a chemical is MOISTURE, MOISTURE, MOISTURE. We offer oils that assist through this entire process the proper way: you can even make the product yourself. See Transition Formula in Chapter 14.

Please note while growing out a relaxer, color or perm (Jeri curl) please request regular Hot Oil treatments offered Rxestoratives Hair and Scalp Wellness Center® or at your salon, or make this treatment yourself. This treatment has remarkable oils that give the hair an immediate different look and feel. The hair becomes soft to the touch with the first treatment. Moisture is key. For more information on how to obtain this and other products: www.rxestoratives.com

RELAXER & COLOR TIPS

PLEASE SEEK THE ADVICE OF A PROFESSIONAL FOR CHEMICAL SERVICES. But IF YOU MUST BE A KITCHEN BEAUTICIAN READ ON.

- ❖ Don't leave relaxer on longer than the directions say you should. Follow the **instructions** on the box.
- ❖ Wash the relaxer out with a conditioner or reconstructor (French Perm is a good reconstructor), follow with Neutralizing Shampoo.
- ❖ Use conditioner after relaxing your hair!
- ❖ Be extra careful when using hair relaxers on children. Keep hair relaxers out of children's reach. (Box relaxers are not the best for hair)
- ❖ It's a good idea to get help with relaxers instead of doing it yourself. This way you are sure to apply and rinse the product from places you can't see.
- ❖ You can protect your scalp by putting petroleum jelly on the scalp before using the relaxer. It prevents the relaxer being absorbed into the scalp. PETROL CHEMICALS DON'T ABORB INTO the SKIN petrol chemicals are from gasoline crude oil (petrol is gasoline)
- ❖ Don't scratch your head or brush your hair before you use a relaxer.

- Do not shampoo hair five (5) days prior to relaxing the hair.
- How often should I relax my hair?
  - Straightening or using a Relaxer too often can lead to damage over processed hair. Ask your hairdresser for advice, because different products on the market have different directions and instructions. According to some hairdressers, every six to eight weeks is common, but this depends on the product. It also depends on your hair, and how fast your hair grows.
    - It's best to do a relaxer only when necessary not every time you go to the salon! Most stylist offer a "spot perm" to give a finish look to the hairstyle- the downside of this are the edges. Look at people edges to see what a "spot perm" long term does to the hairline and edges.
- Can I dye and relax my hair at the same time?
  - You are more likely to damage your hair if you use both permanent hair dye and a relaxer on the same day.
  - If you color your relaxed hair, some hairdressers say you should use a rinse or demi-color. It causes less damage than a permanent dye. Also by using a demi-color with ten Volume will be safe enough to use the same day as a relaxer. Let the color sit on the hair for no more than 15-20 minutes Wash the color out with conditioner then rinse NO SHAMPOO.
  - Refer to product directions and talk to your hairdresser because different relaxers have different instructions.
  - Perform a deep conditioner when you choose to color and relax the hair on the same day.

CHAPTER 6

Food, Vitamins and Nutrients for Hair Growth

Genesis 9:3 - Every moving thing that liveth shall be meat for you; even as the green herb have I given you all things. KJV

No matter how often hair is washed, conditioned and brushed, essential hair vitamins are necessary for hair to be healthy. Hair growth vitamins, and nutrients promotes hair growth. Luster and sheen can be purchased in nearly every pharmacy, grocery store, or vitamin and health food near you or shop online.

Hair consists mainly of proteins called keratins (90%) and the other 10% is water, so if you adopt a healthy lifestyle your body and hair will benefit from it. Gently massaging the scalp with oils and drinking plenty of fluids will help keep the hair follicles (producing hair growth) on the scalp stimulated. Combined with a supplement of liquid silica, a protein and a vitamin rich diet will enable the body to produce strong hair and keep it looking healthy and shiny.

Eating more protein will help make hair thicker if you have very fine or thin hair.

Diet for Hair Loss

A diet that contains whole foods, particularly consuming the outer skin of plants such as green and red peppers, sweet potatoes or regular baked potato, cucumbers and sprouts can offer natural strength to hair because they are rich silica a well-known mineral for hair care. Foods that are high in iron, such as lean meats, are another important food for people with a known iron deficiency.

From this point, this section is for MEN -TO PAGE 64. Women with thinning hair and hair loss, shows there are signs of internal issues going on. One main sign of internal problems is in the gastrointestinal tract. This clearly would be a sign of insufficient stomach acids, in the stomach. It could also be a deficiency of mineral such as: zinc, copper, protein and other necessary nutrients needed for healthy hair. Just by adding or drinking acidophilus milk or taking two acidophilus tablets before, after or in-between meals (four to six tablets per day) for two months may curve the hair loss issue.

By adopting a low-fat diet in **males** this can possibly assist or even slow down the thinning, balding process. Scientists suggest that the **male** pattern baldness is linked to increased testosterone levels during puberty. A high-fat, meat-based diet raises testosterone levels, and that may unfavorably affect hair follicles.

Nutritional Supplements, Vitamins & Herbs

Saw Palmetto - Saw palmetto oil is an accepted treatment for benign prostate hyperplasia in men. It appears to interact with various sex hormones, including dihydrotestoseteron (DHT). DHT is produced from testosterone by enzyme 5-alpha-reductase. Like most enzymes, it can be inhibited. There has been great medical interest in substances that have the potential for inhibiting 5-alpha-reductase, and thereby preventing or treating benign prostate hyperplasia. Theoretically, saw palmetto could have also be used to block DHT and prevent hair loss. Saw palmetto is believed to have a similar mechanism of action to the anti-androgenic drug finasteride (Propecia), which has been used in low doses for hair loss.

L-Phenylalanine, Folic acid, Biotin, Vitamin B5, Para-Amino benzoic acid (PABA), and silica are supplements that may help maintain the thickness and color.

By checking your daily consumption of Zinc whether through tablets or liquid (liquid is always best) make sure you take 30 mg or higher for more than three months or more and this can change a deficiency of copper, and lower copper levels will result in less hair loss.

Speak to a health care practitioner before starting any supplement regimen. Consuming too much copper can be harmful to the body and incite unwanted issues. Having a diet complete with liquid silica, calcium and iron, will help reduce and even prevent hair loss. Eating seaweed type veggies are a good source of minerals and beneficial in reversing and even stopping hair loss. Raw steel or regular oats provide silica. Dried fruits and cherry juice are rich sources of iron

In a **male** trial case study, by adding Silica to the shampoo help prevent baldness, stimulated healthier hair growth and almost 100% offered beautiful shine, luster and gave strength to each strand. Scientists in another country believed that they have successfully stopped/slowed down hair loss; based on a case study that was performed- they believed that by further adding liquid silica to the males shampoo it reduced their hair loss. This can be taken internally or applied externally to regrow already lost hair.

If you have a dysfunctional thyroid whether it is hyper or hypo, the best approach is to eat foods rich in iodine and foods high in vitamin A. Eating vegetables for instance like spinach or carrots, any type of cold-pressed seed oils such as flax, pumpkin seed or even walnut and consuming sea salt on daily basis. By eating peanuts, pine nuts, soy beans, also tofu, turnips, mustard, cabbage, and millet if there is a deficiency of iodine then use this to reverse the issue. But DO NOT overdose on Vitamin. A.

The following are minerals and vitamins necessary for healthy hair growth. By sticking to a regimen with these suggested food items having healthy long strong hair is conceivable.

Since the hair, as we mentioned earlier, is comprised of mostly protein, eating a diet high in protein is recommended. By eating calf's liver, wheat germ, a few tablespoons of lecithin, brewer's yeast this offers a beneficial nutrient of protein.

Protein, found mainly in cold water fish such as salmon. Crab is a luscious remedy for thinning, lack of luster, and weak hair. To infuse elasticity back into limp tresses, go for California rolls and crab cakes. Crab meat is a great source of copper, necessary for healthy melanin production. Add more shellfish on your menu, your mane and eyebrows will be thicker and shinier than ever.

- Minerals Copper & Zinc found in red meats, bran flakes, cocoa, legumes, Silica.
- Vitamins, Biotin, found in liver, eggs, nuts (walnuts) & carrots. Walnuts prevent hair from breaking off, drying out, and turning white. Experts agree that these tasty treats imbue the scalp with oxygen and nutrients. What's more; by preventing cholesterol from blocking arteries they guarantee a healthy blood flow to the head.
- EFAs, Flaxseed Oil, Primrose Oil, and Salmon Oil are good sources they improve hair texture. Prevents dry, brittle hair. Information located at www.fashionlines.com

Vitamins/Nutrients that Prevent Hair Loss

The following vitamins will stimulate and feed the hair follicle to encourage it to produce hair growth, and can be helpful when experiencing hair loss. Vitamins for hair loss can be found in many different vegetables and other foods that we eat every day. Taking a vitamin supplement providing nutrients for hair growth can be a solution for people with a busy lifestyle and provide additional vitamins to nurture health and hair.

- Iron (found in red meats and leafy vegetables such as spinach, kale, broccoli, bok choy). Avoid foods that decrease iron absorption: Tannin beverages: Black & Green Tea at breakfast cut iron absorption in half, Milk Oxalates found in chocolates, Swiss chard & rhubarb.

- Vitamin C (at least 1,000 mg), found in citrus fruits, especially lime. Helps absorption of iron.
- B vitamins, especially Biotin.
- Silica promotes healthy hair, less wrinkles, beautiful nails, great for bones & joints.
- Zinc (12 mg for women, 15 mg for men) will stimulate the blood circulation and encourages follicles to grow hair.

Supplements

Hair growth supplements are available throughout the world and by using the right ones can support boost healthy hair growth. Consuming vitamins and supplements can never replace eating a healthy diet. Hair vitamins and supplements and nutrients can be found in the following vitamin supplements listed below:

- Vitamin B3 Niacin for the health & growth of hair (50 mg 3 times daily)
- Vitamin B5 Pantothenic acid (100mg 3 times daily)
- Vitamin B6 (50 mg taken daily) Men deficient in this vitamin often lose their hair.
- Vitamin E increases oxygen uptake, which improves circulation to the scalp. (400 IU daily and slowly increase to 800-1000 IU daily)
- Silica improves regrowth & strength of the hair follicle (suggested BioSil found at health food stores use six drops in juice first thing in the morning)
- Vitamin C daily improves scalp circulation. Maintains capillaries that carry blood to the follicles. (3,000-10,000 mg daily)
- Magnesium- Controls thinning and thickening of hair (take with

Biotin/BioSil)

- Zinc and Sulfur- Stimulates hair growth by enhancing immune function. (50-100 mg daily)
- Inositol is vital for hair growth (100mg twice daily)
- Coenzyme Q10 Improves scalp circulation. Increases tissue oxygenation. It's great for heart health also. (60 mg daily)
- L-Cysteine & L-Methionine: Two amino acids believed to improve quality, texture and growth of hair. They prevent hair from falling out. (500 mg each twice daily on an empty stomach)

NOTE: It is wise to always check with your doctor before taking supplements, as he or she will be able to advice you about the best options for you. A dietician, nutritionist or nutritional consultant, can help you compile a diet plan providing the necessary minerals and vitamins to provide to sufficient amounts of nutrients for hair growth. Exercise will stimulate the circulation of blood throughout the entire body so the scalp will also benefit from this, promoting hair growth. Do not take all supplements at the same time. See practitioner for proper dosage.

Avoid crash diets. They stress the body and the effects appear in all the body's systems. Remember that hair is nothing more than a-keratin protein (90% with the remaining 10% being water.) A low protein diet can cause the hair to thin and will certainly slow its growth.

Sources for Getting These Nutrients Naturally

The best natural supply for vitamins mineral and nutrients to be the most effective for hair growth and for the benefit of the body is to maintain a healthy diet, incorporate fresh cold water fish (salmon), consume nuts, fresh fruits (vitamin C) and eating lean meats (zinc) and iron. A diet compiled of the necessary food will not only make hair grow and look better, but will also ensure stronger longer healthy looking hair, nails and skin. When preparing vegetables, it is important to prepare them quickly and to reduce cooking times to a minimum, as overcooking vegetables will reduce the amount of vitamins and nutrients that they contain.

It should be everyone's goal to eat at least two (2) citrus fruits per day or even drinking something citrus like Orange juice, Grapefruit juice. This fruit (often provides a high dose of vitamins for hair loss) even by adding lime juice to drinks or salad dressings will provide a high dose of vitamin C as well. Out of all the citrus fruits the lime has the highest dose of vitamin C.

Due to the fact, that our choices in food has greatly deteriorated everyone young or old can benefit from taking a multivitamin or mineral supplements, its best to take them in liquid for quick consumption.

The B and E vitamins are good for your hair as are zinc, sulfur, kelp and magnesium. Also, make sure your multivitamin includes biotin and liquid silica. To get more B vitamins from your diet, eat beans, peas, carrots, cauliflower, soybeans, bran, nuts preferably walnuts (as mentioned earlier they are most beneficial for the hair and skin, blood vessels cholesterol), and eggs. Avocados, nuts, seeds, and olive oil contain the E vitamins.

Avoid foods that are full of grease and fat. They will disrupt your digestive system and potentially make your scalp and hair very oily. Reduce your consumption of salt because it tends to raise your blood pressure and distress blood circulation to your scalp. As this relates to male pattern baldness avoid food that are greasy food and full of salt, this affects male and female high blood pressure. Avoid at all cost processed foods: they are full of chemical additives and have unnecessary preservative ingredients that does not agree with our bodies, plus lessen your intake of fast foods as well. But do eat a well-balanced diet with plenty of fruits and vegetables and a lot of protein which is found in meat is your best bet when desiring long beautiful healthy hair.

Most times we ask, "what do I want to eat today?" The next time this thought is bouncing around in your mind think on these things, foods that are beneficial for your hair and skin:

For healthy hair, your diet must contain a balanced quantity of vitamins, antioxidants, minerals and proteins. Without Omega Capital -369 fatty acids, hair is often dry and lifeless. Foods rich in biotin, copper, zinc, selenium, and PABA may promote hair growth & slow hair loss.

MELONS

Melons are great for flushing toxins out of the body first thing in the morning. Just by eating 12 pieces of melons in the morning will help to flush out the rest of the toxins out of your body.

Melons come in many varieties ---- the watermelon the red melon, the yellow melon the Cantaloupe and the Honeydew the green melon. Melon contains Vitamin C and are high in potassium content, with traces of Vitamin B complex. They help to flush out toxins and waste materials from the kidneys.

GRAPEFRUIT

Compared to other citrus fruits, (oranges, lemons, limes, tangerines) the grapefruit is loaded with tons of Vitamin C. There is not a large amount of vitamins B, E, and K complex, but enough minerals, phosphorus, potassium and even calcium. Just by drinking this fruit, and by adding iron-rich foods, the Vitamin C found in this fruit will aid in the absorption of iron.

Grapefruit helps in preventing colds it strengthens the capillary walls and helps in the overall healing rejuvenating process in the body. But the high pectin content of grapefruit juice interferes with the absorption of dietary fat, so people with weak digestive systems should try to avoid it.

DARK LEAFY GREEN VEGGIES

Dark leafy green veggies are high in iron (Collard Greens, Mustard Greens, Spinach, Asparagus) and drink fresh fruit and /or vegetable juice at least once per day. Science indicates this natural pigment found in dark green, leafy vegetables may be linked to the promotion of healthy hair and skin.

Having proper nourishment for your body and hair is very important. Just like your body, hair needs a balanced, nutritious diet to grow, stay supple, shimmering and youthful-looking. Eat easily digestible healthy foods at regular intervals for healthy hair. A diet that is lacking in basic nutritional building blocks such as protein can cause problems with hair growth, and depending on the severity of the dietary intake, can cause problems with hair loss.

EFA help sebaceous glands to control dryness and brittle hair and improve its texture. Such as Flax Seed Oil, Wheat Germ & Walnuts.

VITAMINS AND ANTIOXIDANTS

Vitamins and antioxidants: certain fruits & vegetables are loaded with hair growing vitamins and nutrients. Combine various fruits and vegetables for the required dose of vitamins your body need.

Vitamins B: It is necessary for growth of healthy hair. This vitamin is beneficial for hair growth because it helps in the formation of red blood cells. Red blood cells carry oxygen throughout the body even the scalp causing our us to growth healthy hair. So, B vitamins are important very for the health and growth of the hair. Leading Food Sources of Vitamin B: Beans, Peas, Carrots, Cauliflower, Soy Beans (men be aware that soy is a high carrier of estrogen), Nutritional Yeast, Bran, Nuts, and Eggs. For best results take with the other B vitamin mentioned earlier.

Vitamin C: For improved circulation of nutrients to the scalp area.

COPPER

Copper found in Mushrooms, sunflower seeds, most nuts, any type of seafood, coco and legumes is an essential ingredient in melanin. This is where we get our color from the pigment of our skin hair so forth. With Copper combined with Zinc, both are usually found in the same food sources having healthy hair should not be an issue.

Vitamin E: Helps increase oxygen intake and improves circulation, improving hair quality and growth. Highest food form of Vitamin. E is found in Wheat Germ.

Minerals: Iodine found in kelp, yogurt (low fat), cow's milk, boiled eggs, strawberries and Mozzarella cheese, are the best source of this mineral.

GRAINS AND NUTS

Grains and nuts in Ezekiel Bread found in the frozen section at grocery stores is a great source of healthier alternate for bread.

Protein and iron: Lean meats, beans and legumes for protein and green leafy vegetables for iron. Make sure you combine foods with Vitamin C in the same meal for better absorption of Iron. Avoid taking iron supplements. You should get your Iron from food sources. Leading Food Sources of Iron: Oysters, lean red meat, liver, poultry, tuna, Iron-fortified cereals, whole grains, dried beans, eggs, dried fruit, dark green leafy vegetables, wheat, millet, oats, brown rice, Lima beans, soy beans, dried beans and peas, kidney beans, almonds, Brazil nuts, prunes, raisins, apricots, broccoli, spinach, kale, collards, asparagus, dandelion greens.

WATER

A great healthy hair tip is to drink plenty of water especially one with a high pH (8.8) to keep yourself well hydrated. Approximate half your body weight or 8-10. 8 oz a day is the minimum quantity. Water helps to flush toxins from the body toxins that leads to hair loss, or even compromises our immune system

Doctors recommend use of Soy products especially for women because it has the most needed hormone that women can truly benefit from (Estrogen) and multi-vitamins. By adding theses supplements into your diet will not only boost your health but also will make your hair healthier and more elasticized (causing less breakage and hair loss).

Avoid the following as they can reduce blood flow to the scalp, cause excess stress and promote hair loss:

- Alcohol
- Smoking
- Eating highly processed foods (Fried food, most snack foods, cookies, cakes, candies)
- Overeating

OMEGA-3•6•9 FATTY ACIDS
Omega-3•6•9 may help reduce flaking dandruff and itching scalp, as well as eczema and psoriasis of the scalp. Leading Food Sources of Omega-3•6•9 Fatty Acids: Salmon, Tuna, Trout.

PABA
PABA known as Para-Amino Benzoic Acid has been documented to protect hair follicles and prevent hair loss. By reversing the deficiency of PABA some studies show that this may also be useful for restoring gray hair back to its natural color. Leading Food Sources of PABA: Rice, brown, Mushrooms, Eggs, Milk, Oysters

SELENIUM
This is a very important mineral that our bodies need for healthy hair and just to be healthy period. This mineral is also an antioxidant it cleans up dangerous free radical that might in the body. This is like a having a boxer in your body that wins every round. It also works well with certain hormones in our bodies. This mineral fights off cancerous cells, helps prevent impaired vision, reverse hair loss, guard again heart attacks and so much more. Research suggests that this mineral may enhance healthy hair growth.

Leading Food Sources of Selenium: Rice, brown, Chicken, Wheat, Shrimp, Sunflower seeds, Tuna, Brazil nuts, Eggs

ZINC
Zinc is very beneficial for people who have brittle or thinning hair, if it is due to an under active thyroid this mineral is a must to consume. It also stimulates hair growth by improving immunity. You can get enough of zinc and iron from green vegetables.

Leading Food Sources of Zinc: Barley, Oysters, Crab, Chicken, Wheat, Lamb, Beef, Turkey. A fortified breakfast of cereal will provide your body will all other required nutrients. Eat easily digestible simple food at regular intervals. Do not over eat.

Nutrition: Vitamins and Minerals

With an inadequate diet hair loss is inevitable, the B vitamins, minerals and amino acids are of most importance especially for healthy hair growth.

Two healthy foods/supplement suggestions are to make sure you are consuming enough B vitamins and drinking an adequate amount of milk (low-fat or regular). Milk contains casein and it also has a protein known as whey protein and it carries lipids. Proteins and lipids together make the roots of hair stronger. Calcium boosts healthy growing hair and is known to prevent hair loss. Vitamins A, B6, and biotin with potassium causes the hair to have a beautiful sheen to it.

B vitamins are important if you desire healthy long growing hair. Foods rich in B vitamins include *beans, peas, carrots, cauliflower, soy beans, nutritional yeast, bran, nuts and eggs.* Take a vitamin B complex and supplement it with the following additional B vitamins for best results.

- Vitamin B3 (niacin)
- Vitamin B 5 (pathothenol)
- Vitamin B 6 (pyridoxine-an amino acid)
- Biotin
- Folic Acid
- Magnesium *Sulfur* Zinc
- Inositol
- Raw thymus
- L-Cysteine and L-Methionine

There are specific necessary amino acids that control the thickness and thinning of the hair. Magnesium is necessary for having healthy strong long hair. When B vitamins that are beneficial for hair growth are combined with this mineral the hair is completely restored-if hair loss is the clients' issue.

Following a strict regimen of vitamins and supplements will result in the stimulation of hair growth. When men show signs of hair loss or receding hair line this may be a sign of vitamin B6 deficiency. ***Note: a medical doctor is qualified to diagnosis this deficiency not a cosmetologist.***

In the mean- time, if they were to add folic acid and B6 their daily dietary routine they may or could have slowed down this process and even reverse it.

****Caution when consuming vitamin A (100,000 IU) in excess this may result in hair loss. The positive side to this vitamin is when you stop consuming the vitamin the hair loss is reversed.*

There are natural ingredients (oils) that are known to improve hair textures and prevents brittle dull dry hair they are:

- Evening Primrose Oil
- Flaxseed
- Omega 6
- Salmon Oil

Vitamin Dosages for Hair Growth

- B Vitamins
- Vitamin B3 (niacin) - 50 mg 3 times daily.
- Pantothenic acid (vitamin B5) -100 mg 3 times daily.
- Pyridoxine (vitamin B6) -50 mg 3 times daily.

Biotin

The importance of Biotin for hair health is necessary. Its beneficial for hair and skin and for several men it has been known to prevent hair loss and thinning. With dietary habits that are high in this mineral noticeable hair growth is evident. Food high in this mineral is everyday regular eaten foods. They are: brewer's yeast, brown rice, bulgur, green peas, lentils, oats, soybeans, sunflower seeds, and walnuts. You can also use hair care products containing Biotin.

Dosage: 50 mg 3 times daily.

Coenzyme Q10

Improves scalp circulation. Increases the oxygen in our tissues. Great for a heathy heart and improves skin elasticity.

Dosage: Take 60 mg daily.

Iron

Acts as a stimulant for hair growth. To absorb Iron, vitamin C it vital for hair growth

Dosage: 20 mg (women with menstrual cycle), for men 10 mg daily.

Inositol

Inositol is vital for hair growth. It helps to strengthen the roots or follicles.

Dosage: 100 mg twice daily.

L-Cysteine and L-methionine

Both amino acids improve the texture of hair and allows for the hair grow. May also stop hair from falling out.

Dosage: 500 mg each twice daily, and on an empty stomach.[6]

Vitamin C

Vitamin C taken with irons is beneficial for improving scalp circulation and acts as a stimulant.

Dosage: 90-200 mg daily. The recommended daily intake of Vitamin C is 90 mg but to address a deficiency in the vitamin, supplementation with 200 mg daily is advised.

Vitamin E

Vitamin E improves circulation which in turn increases oxygen to the scalp. It improves the health and growth of hair. The growth/health of our

---

[6] http://www.holistic-online.com/remedies/hair/hair_loss-diet.htm

hair is connected to our immune system and having a healthy immune system may stimulate hair growth.

Dosage: Start with 400 IU daily and slowly increase to 800-1,000 IU daily.

Raw Thymus glandular

This herb works with the body thymus gland, it stimulates the immune function and improves the function of other glands.

Dosage: 500 mg daily. **Not for children!

Zinc

Zinc is a mineral can help to restore thinning hair and help improve hair growth. Zinc helps with cell reproduction. Helps the body absorb iron and other vitamins. Works with the immune system as well. This mineral is needed for the prevention of hair loss.

Dosage: 50-100 mg daily. Do not exceed this amount Vitamins

Vitamin A must be obtained via food and supplements. This vitamin known as retinol (for the eyes) and helps your eyes adjust to light, its known to receive beta carotene, from orange fruits and vegetables. The beneficial of this vitamin is it is an antioxidant the neutralize free radicals in the body, these type of free radicals causes cellular and tissue damage. The body can produce vitamins from food (for example, eating carrots, pumpkin, broccoli turns into Vitamin A forms beta carotene). Some other vitamins have special area in the body where this vitamin is produced for example Vitamin K in produced a microorganism found in the gut and Vitamin D is produced by the sun

Each vitamin has a recommended daily allowance which should be adhered to for optimal health. We may find it in our food and if not we take supplements.

NOTE: Conditions Associated with Vitamin Deficiencies

There are debilitating deficiencies that is associated with every vitamin. For example, **Vitamin A** deficiency is related to night-blindness; **B3 (Niacin)** with pellagra (deficiency of niacin); vitamin C with scurvy; and vitamin D with rickets.
However, vitamin deficiencies rarely cause debilitating ailment. In fact, each vitamin deficiency can be detected early with signs that make us go and see our physician. Like if you are low in iron you are experiencing fatigue, light headiness.

With certain deficiencies from vitamins specific signs of a deficiency will be evident, especially with hair loss. Hair will be all over the floor, the scalp may become extremely itchy, tender and soar. This would be sign of needing silica, or Omega oils, B vitamins, but again a doctor would be able to confirm this with a blood test.

Hair and skin are external and my belief is what goes in is what comes out. If there are internal deficiencies it should be treated internally. If your hair starts falling out begin to trace when this was the first sign you noticed the hair falling out so you can be able to accurately determine the best course of action. Was there something traumatic going on. Did you start a new exercise regimen? Did you start taking new medication. Had surgery that required anesthesia? If the answer is no to these questions, then vitamin deficiency may be another consideration.

See chart on the next page.

VITAMIN DAILY DOSAGE	QUICK REFERENCE
Vitamin A or Retinol	**- 1-5 mg**
Vitamin B	**- 2 mg (B6), 0.5 mg (Biotin), 25 - 50 mg (para-amino**

VITAMIN DAILY DOSAGE	QUICK REFERENCE
	benzoic acid
Vitamin C or Ascorbic Acid	**- 75 - 200 mg**
Vitamin D or Calciferol	**- 5 micrograms**
Vitamin E or Tocopherol	**- 10 - 30 mg**

Diet

Make sure you are aware that you need to follow a healthy, well balanced diet, to avoid consequences which, may lead to hair loss. Having metabolism issues will lead to vitamin deficiencies as well, most of the time a poor diet is the major contributor.

The most important vitamins beneficial to healthy hair are vitamins A, C, D, and E. Several people are not familiar with the benefits of vitamins for hair loss, and the vital role vitamins play in our health status. It is wise to become knowledgeable with the various vitamins required for health.

Vitamin A

There is such a vitamin known as the moisture vitamin. This vitamin helps to keep moisture in the hair. Vitamin A helps. in the discharge of sebum (oil) into the scalp. We need sebum (oil) to have healthy scalp and hair. Taking Vitamin, A will cause the hair from brittle and being dry. Take caution when using this vitamin, it is an antioxidant. If you over use this vitamin the opposite is it will lead to hair loss called Hypervitaminosis A.

Vitamin B

Has over 7 other B vitamins that all perform in different. This vitamin is not a single vitamin this vitamin has unique chemically derived characteristics in some food sources. The following vitamins beneficial for hair and skin care are:

- Vitamin B3 (niacin)
- Vitamin B 5 (pantothenol)
- Vitamin B 6 (pyridoxine-an amino acid)
- Vitamin B7 (Biotin)
- Vitamin B9 (Folic acid)
- Magnesium *Sulfur* Zinc
- Inositol
- Raw thymus
- L-Cysteine and L-Methionine

With an inadequate diet, hair loss is inevitable, the B vitamins, minerals and amino acids are of most importance especially for healthy hair growth. Two healthy foods suggested to eat and to and ensure that you are getting enough B vitamins are milk (low or non-fat is best to avoid getting too much unhealthy fat in your diet) and egg yolks.

B vitamins are important for the health and growth of the hair. Foods rich in B vitamins include: **avocado,** ***bran,*** **beef,** ***beans, carrots, cauliflower, dates, eggs,*** **lamb,** ***nuts, nutritional yeast, peas, poultry, salmon, soy beans, tuna and trout, watermelon.***

Take a vitamin B complex and supplement it with the following additional B vitamins for best results.

There are specific necessary amino acids that control the thickness and thinning of the hair. Magnesium is necessary for having healthy strong long hair. When B vitamins that are beneficial for hair growth are combined with this mineral the hair is completely restored-if hair loss is the clients' issue. Following a strict regimen of vitamins and supplements will result in the stimulation of hair growth. When men show signs of hair loss or receding hair line this may be a sign of vitamin B6 deficiency. ***Note: a medical doctor is qualified to diagnosis this deficiency not a cosmetologist.***

In the mean- time, if you were to add folic acid and B6 your daily dietary routine you may or could have slowed down this process and even reverse it.

Having a deficiency of this vitamin in our bodies will tend to lead to serious health problems and possibly create a chain reaction with a combination of other vitamins that are also deficient. For this vitamin to truly be effective high consumptions of this vitamin is necessary, via food is always best.

Vitamin C
or L-ascorbic acid is known to very important to having healthy skin. This vitamin help develop collagen and this is what the skin needs and consist of. Therefore, **Vitamin C** deficiency will lead to scurvy, the manifestation of not enough collage in the skin is skin becomes weak.

In addition, as this pertains to hair care Vi**tamin C** is known produce an amino acid known as tyrosine in the body, and this amino acid gives strength to hair strands and nourish the cells of hair follicles. When there is a deficiency of **Vitamin C,** scurvy and the shedding of hair will be present.

Also, a recent study determined that using a Vitamin C supplement would cause the hair to grow back if it had fallen out. The supplement had the ability to stop a gene in the papills cells that caused a blockage of androgenic cell of the hair follicles-meaning instead of the hair growing it would not grow but fall out. But when the supplement was taken the hair would start growing again.

Vitamin D
Most beneficial for the entire body especially the hair and scalp and vital

for the hair follicles. Its promising in absorbing calcium. This is one of only vitamins that requires sunlight to synthesize vitamin D. This vitamin will cause hair loss if there is a deficiency during the hair growth cycle. This is also a sign of deficiency in this vitamin, what occurs is there is a lack of calcium absorption and hair loss soon follows.
There is a plus in reversing this deficiency, getting more sunlight first thing in the morning and eating or taking supplements or drinking fortified dairy products

Vitamin E
By taking vitamin E there is an increase in blood circulation because oxygen is provided for the hair follicles. To have healthy hair follicles oxygen is needed not only to breathe (live) but the health of the scalp because this help to regenerate the follicles causing them to grow. The deficiency of this vitamin and other vitamin will allow the opposite to happen.

Pantothenic Acid also known as **Calcium Pantothenate,** If, you don't like gray hair then adding this vitamin to your regimen can reverse gray hair and even cause hair loss to be reversed or the hair grows back darker. This vitamin can be obtained through your diet.

Flaxseed oil salmon oil and primrose oil, in addition to vitamins helps to improve the quality and texture of hair and it aids in having brittle dry hair. There are many other nutrients you should have in your diet to promote healthy hair growth.

When your diet includes valuable vitamins and other nutrients you need for your overall good health, you can be guaranteed that having healthier hair and preventing hair loss.

14 Vitamins That Help Hair Loss

Having to deal with hair loss often can be a hassle. This is an issue that affects millions of people throughout the world. Hair loss can be treated or addressed just having a basic change in diet and lifestyle can address the problem. There are specific vitamins for men for hair loss that differ a little for women to avoid the loss of hair. By having adequate vitamins nutrients and supplements which people are not clearly aware of hair loss can be avoided. By incorporating the necessary vitamins, nutrients which are found in various foods, fruits and vegetables not only will our lifestyle be better but our bodies will be in a healthier state. What goes in is what comes out. Healthy eating, healthy living and healthy hair.

Note: it's best to find as many vitamins/nutrients in liquid form when necessary. Liquid enters the blood stream faster than capsules and pills. Capsules and pills must enter the digestive system first then filter its way into the blood stream...just something to think about.

 # 1 - Amino Acids Hair Loss

When combined with other vitamins nutrients and amino acids hair loss can be treated. The non-essential amino acids and essential amino acids are best for treating thinning hair.

- ❖ **Methionine**: an excellent source of sulfur and this is very strong antioxidant.
- ❖ **Cysteine**: an amino acid that increases hair significantly this considered a non-essential amino acid.
- ❖ **Cystine**: is used to treat thinning hair this non-essential amino acid promotes hair growth as well.
- ❖ **Tyrosine**: another non-essential amino acid that is used to treat many health problems, including hair loss.

 # 2 – Vitamin A for Hair Loss

Vitamin A is used for producing hair and scalp oil. Carrots are needed to produce hair/scalp oil. Without adequate sebum, our hair gets dry and brittle, dandruff and a thick scalp will develop, both of which can be aggravating but it can be treated. After the hair has prolonged dryness it begins to break thin out and can lead to permanent hair loss

Vitamin A is an antioxidant which can be obtained from any orange colored fruit or vegetables such as mangos, oranges, carrots, sweet potatoes, squash, and liver.

 # 3 – Vitamin B for Hair Loss

Having a healthy hemoglobin is necessary for having or treating hair loss. Hemoglobin carries oxygen to the scalp and to the red blood cells. There are more various B vitamins but there one that is most beneficial is Vitamin B6 known as amino benzoic acid and Biotin and inositol.
Vitamin B can be obtained from oats, eggs, poultry, beef, beans peas, seafood bananas, potatoes and non-fat milk.

 # 4 - Beta Sitosterol Hair Loss

This is a natural plant extract, mineral that can be found to be most effective supplement for male pattern baldness, hair loss and thinning. This plant is full of nutrients most beneficial for having healthy hair and for encouraging new hair growth. As of date there no recorded side effects when using this plant/supplement.

 # 5 – Hair Loss Biotin

Food for your hair is what **Biotin** is known for. This supplement Biotin plays a huge role in hair loss. For healthy hair adding Biotin your daily supplement regimen will play an important role in keeping hair healthy.
This vitamin/mineral can be found in liver and eggs. That's why when people start dieting and leave out the yoke from the egg they begin to **experience hair loss. Its better drink (liquid) vitamin than to take them** (pills, capsules) for best results. When taking/drinking/consuming Biotin add magnesium to the diet as well. Certain minerals need magnesium for the body to absorb the mineral.

 # 6 – Vitamin C for Hair Loss

Oranges is high in this vitamin. Vitamin C produces collagen which is important in having healthy hair. Vitamin C helps to avoid many documented health issues. It's also good in helping preventing cold especially the flu. When taking **Vitamin C**, the absorption of iron is found in fruit and vegetables in the daily diet. Citrus fruits are loaded with Vitamin C as is berries: strawberries, blueberries, green and red peppers mango and guava.

 # 7 – Vitamin D for Hair Loss

Hair loss and rickets are two health issues associated with a lack of **Vitamin D**. It is involved in the health of hair follicles. Fatty acids like Omega 3, 6, 9 play a role in the body's production of **Vitamin D**. Without enough essential fatty acids, the body is not able to produce enough **Vitamin D**, which leads to a deficiency that may cause psoriasis and a flaky scalp.

 # 8 -- Vitamin E for Hair Loss

Safflower oil – for good blood circulation in the hair and scalp consuming **Vitamin E** it's for helping to absorb oxygen.

You can find **Vitamin E** in several vegetable oils, corn, safflower, soybean oil, nuts, leafy green vegetables. Again, as mentioned earlier its best to ingest **Vitamin E** rather than use it as a topical solution or take it as a capsule or vitamin. There is more benefits this way. **Vitamin E** is important for healthy hair growth. Eating avocados, nuts, seeds, and olive oil on a regular basis. Encourages hair growth.

 # 9 -- Folic Acid Hair Loss

This vitamin plays a valuable role in preventing hair loss. Eating foods that have folic acid helps to decrease and even prevent hair loss or thinning hair. This is most beneficial for people who are genetically predisposed to hair loss or baldness.

Folic acid can be found in steamed asparagus raw chickpeas, frozen peas, cooked lentils, papaya and collard greens and other green leafy vegetables.

The benefits of folic acid are it supports the tissue growth and helps the cells work correctly. Folic acid helps hair follicles and the scalp to function well. With folic acid, the hair and follicles can grow healthy hair.

- **Folic acid** regenerates cells that grow hair.
- **Folic acid** consistently helps the body increase the circulation. Healthy circulation supports skin cells and hair follicles that generates healthy hair and develops beautiful skin and develops faster hair growth. [7]

 # 10 -- Grape Seed

Grapeseed can be found in capsule, oil, extract and as noted the best form of use is oil. It is safe to treat hair loss. It helps because it stimulates the hair follicles and begin the reverse of thinning and falling hair. People who suffer from poor dietary habits or who have known genetic disorders or diseases are prone to hair loss. By adding Grapeseed to your daily supplement regimen will begin healthy hair growth. It is also a great detox for the body as well.

 # 11 -- Iron Hair Loss

Iron deficiency can cause hair loss in women, it is important for women to receive this nutrient in abundance. This is also considered an oxidant (it's an addition of oxygen to something….) It's found in many of the foods we eat on a regular basis. This mineral is known to stimulate hair growth, with this nutrient Vitamin C intake is necessary to be able to absorb iron.

---

[7] http://vitanetonline.com/forums

There are three main reasons why women may have iron deficiencies:

- Heavy periods with a lot of bleeding
- Ulcers and inflammations of the stomach- bleeding in the digestive tract
- Loss of blood after giving birth.

Dietary sources of iron include lean red meat, dried fruit, tofu and broccoli.

Since iron is so useful yet toxic at high doses, free iron in the cell is strictly regulated. Instead, iron is found bound to proteins. In this form, iron can be safely used by the body.

Heme is the most popular of these proteins which binds to iron. It is found in the hemoglobin of red blood cells and has the vital function of transporting oxygen and carbon dioxide to and from the lungs and other parts of the body.

For cell metabolism, the body needs iron for oxygen transport. When a lot of blood is lost, there is a severe fall in iron levels which leads to anemia. The human body needs 5 grams of iron in the red blood cells for oxygen throughout the body. Half of the iron is stored in the cells the other half is stored as ferritin in other parts of the body like the bone marrow spleen liver and cells. When these iron levels drop, it takes it from these other sites where iron is stored.

 # 12 -- Inositol Hair Loss

This can be called a sweet herb/mineral, inositol is known to inhibit hair loss. People use this mineral to treat thinning hair in men and women. This is used to help inhibit hair loss and allow healthy hair to grow back. It has anti- oxidant properties that allow the hair follicles to remain healthy. It is also great for reducing cholesterol levels.

There are many delicious ways you can get plenty of inositol in your diet, including *unrefined molasses, raisins, Brewer's yeast, oat flakes, nuts, wheat germ, bananas, beef and pork brain, liver, hearts, brown rice and a variety of vegetables.*

#13 – Omega 3

This is an essential fatty acid (EFA), and it is necessary that we have **Omega-3** acids for healthy hair. The three main nutrients found in **Omega 3**s are ALA (alpha linoleic acid), EPA (ecoisapentaionic acid (pronounced iso-sa-pantic-e-no-ic acid)) and DHA (docosahexaenioc acid (pronounced do-caw-sa-has-ic-e-noic acid). This EFA may be found in various seafood such as albacore, black cod, catfish, clams, halibut, herring, mackerel, salmon, shrimp, trout, tuna and other foods or nuts such as almonds, flax seed and walnuts.

Omega 6 As with Omega 3 Omega 6 this EFA is derived from food, our bodies do not make this fatty acid and it must be obtaining via food. Omega 6 increases the immune response like in cell production, blood clotting but in Omega 3 it's the opposite therefore there is a balance. This fatty acid that is found in Carrier Oils like: Grapeseed Safflower, Soybean and Sunflower these fatty acids encourages hair growth and assist in improving skin conditions like eczema and some scalp conditions. Taken internally when purchased in food grade and externally when applied to the scalp/hair directly.

Omega 9 Getting these omegas is in food is probably food we are eating already. Now to get omega in the hair is another topic to discuss

Quick Tip #1

Most people's hair grows about 5-7 inches per year on average. We all have an estimated 100K strands on our scalp and it is not uncommon to lose 25-100 strands per day. One of the most common causes of hair falling is improper combing, detangling and brushing and the improper use of product.

altogether. Omega 9 controls the loss of water in the hair and it makes the hair softer and malleable. Another tip this fatty acid helps to regulate the bad cholesterol and helps your body's immune function. [8]

Silica for Hair Loss

Silica is one of the most abundant minerals in the earth. It is found in sand, rocks and even dirt. It is almost as abundant in the earth as in the body. Silica is found in our hair, nails, joints, muscles and just about all over the body. This mineral is vital for our health.

The health of your hair depends greatly on your intake of this mineral, in addition to that, the rate at which it grows. African American women spend thousands of dollars on deep conditioning treatments in hopes that they will stimulate hair growth and mend split ends, seldom realizing that it is more about what they put into their hair as opposed to on it, to fix the problem. Silica has been proven to improve hair texture, prevent split ends, and accelerate hair growth.

By having high levels of silica in your body, your hair will have little breakage, have shine, and will grow at a faster rate. But where does one obtain silica? Unfortunately, just as our foods are being compromised with poisons, all types of GMO's in our soil are becoming affected and deficient as well.

Colloidal Silica and Liquid Silica

What's the difference? Colloidal: the size of the mineral-it's very small; tiny enough to pass through cell membranes easily, and it does not need to go thru the digestive process. Liquid: is more concentrated and is used less.[9]

---

[8] http://blackgirllonghair.com

[9] Silica: The mineral your hair cannot go without

Fiji Water

If you are not the type to purchase something which can be generally found in abundance for free, consider this: Fiji has 91 mg of natural colloidal silica per liter (32 oz bottle). Fiji water source in known to come from thru several layers of volcanic rock before it is collected and bottled for use. The higher priced water is due its high mineral content and the way its processed.

CHAPTER 7

Understanding pH

Num 11:5 We remember the fish we used to eat in Egypt — it cost us nothing! — and the cucumbers, the melons, the leeks, the onions, the garlic! CJB

This is for Information Purposes Only
Understanding of Alkaline vs. Acidic
The pH scale is from 0 - 14

0 1 2 3 4 5 6 7 healthy 8 9 10 11 12 13 14

❖ **Understanding pH**

These letters represent how much potential hydrogen is in our bodies. The "H" is always capital because on the Periodic charts this represents Hydrogen. The p is always lowercase because it is describing what the Hydrogen is as it pertains to our bodies.

This measures the acidity or alkalinity of a solution. It is measured on a scale of 0 to 14—the lower the pH the more acidic of the solution and the higher the pH the more alkaline (or base) the solution. If a solution is neither acidic nor alkaline then the pH registers a seven which is neutral. To remain disease free, we should stay neutral.

Water makes up about 70% of our body consumption. The body constantly attempts to maintain a balanced pH. When our bodies are not balanced then the door of illnesses and issues begin. Stay balanced by eating right and drinking the appropriate amount of water for healthy living.

Human blood pH should be marginally alkaline (7.35 - 7.45). Below or above this range indicates there is potential illness or disease, when something is not regular we must investigate to find out "why", to resolve the issue. In the body or on any pH scale 7.0 is always Neutral. There are two regulated balances Acidic and Alkaline: pH below 7.0 is Acidic, pH above 7.0 is Alkaline.

An acidic pH can ensue from, an acidic diet, emotional stress, toxic overload, and/or immune reactions or anything that deprives the cells of oxygen and other important nutrients. We naturally have alkaline minerals within our bodies, but with the excess of acids the body attempts to compensate for it. If the diet does not contain enough minerals to compensate, a buildup of acids in the cells will transpire.

Several major issues begin to occur when the body is acidic; Particularly;

- ❖ A diminution in the body's ability to absorb minerals and other necessary nutrients
- ❖ The cells that produce energy decrease
- ❖ Damaged cells are left unrepaired; the body cannot repair these cells on its on
- ❖ A decline in the body's' ability to detoxify heavy metals
- ❖ Tumorous cells increase
- ❖ The body can't seem it get enough rest so fatigue and illness sets in
- ❖ This is slightly acidic when the blood has a pH of 6.9, but believe it or not this can induce coma and even death.

Diet plays and important role in our bodies being Alkaline or Acidic

Our diet mainly contributes to this condition known as acidosis (an exceptionally acid condition found in the body fluids or tissues.) because it has far too much fat in it. These foods are from processed foods and animal by products as well. Food like meat, eggs and dairy, are very low in alkaline and lean more on the acidic side of the scale, but foods like fresh fruit and vegetables meets the acid goal consumption for the day. In addition, we eat acid producing processed foods such as white flour and white sugar and drink acid producing like coffee and carbonated beverages.

When we get ill we take a lot of medication, which are categorized as acid forming; and we use chemical prone artificial sweeteners like Equal, Sweet 'N Low, NutraSweet and Spoonful. The best way to address this issue is of an acidic body is begin a detox program (see your doctor or Naturopathic Doctor) and change the way we eat and see food.
For a rule of thumb: we should consume at least 60% of alkaline type foods and 40% acidic foods. This will put us on a healthy road of restoration. For people with current health issues the scale is a little different: for optimal health and to be restored to a healthy lifestyle then Alkaline foods should be consumed at least 80% of the diet and 20% acidic foods.

Most green leafy vegetables, fruit beans, peas, spices, seasonings, herbs, lentils, and nuts are found to be alkaline; Acid forming foods are known to be eggs, fish grains, legumes, meat and poultry. Believe it or not fats and sugar even starches are neutral, mainly because the do not have sulfur or minerals in them. But again, eating too much of this will lead to weight gain, this is why I stress for you to find the balance in everything you do and eat.

Shifting Your pH Toward Alkaline

When consuming food be aware that food leave behind their own what I call "DNA" (trace that it's been here)- based on how much you eat determines whether you have a high content of acid prone foods in your diet which in turns, leaves traces of sulfur phosphate or alkaline prone foods and likewise will leave traces of calcium, magnesium and or potassium.
If you need help in adjusting your body pH use the chart below as a reference. The scale range from seven Acidic to 14 Alkaline. Below on the scale seven down to zero is Low on Oxygen and seven up to 14 is alkaline. A body that is acidic is prone to illnesses. Keep the body as balanced as possible.

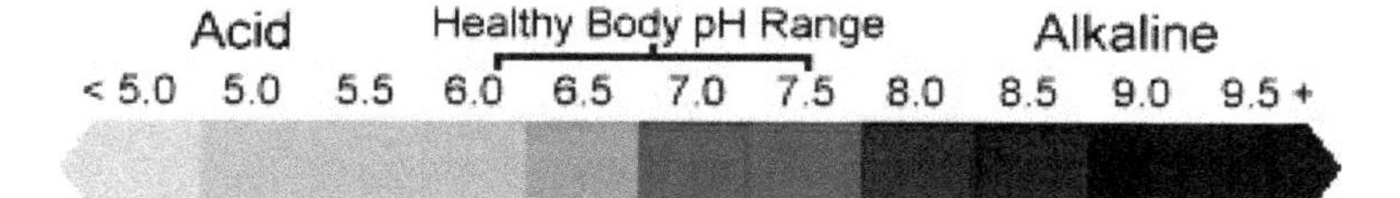

❖ Use pH strips to test your Body's Acidity or Alkalinity: (these can be purchased at Health food stores, Vitamin shops or online (Amazon).

It is highly recommended to test your pH levels to determine if your body's pH needs immediate attention. We are testing body fluids like our urine and saliva. Use the appropriate type of strips that when you open the container they are sealed. Follow the directions on the packaging for accurate readings. In the morning, if your urinary pH reading is between 6.0 to 6.5 and in the evenings the readings are between 6.5 and 7.0, your body is functioning within a healthy range. If your saliva stays between 6.5 and 7.5 all day, your body is functioning within a healthy range. The optimal time to test your pH is about one hour before a meal and two hours after a meal. Test your pH two days a week.

NOTE: This chart **does not** regulate or discuss your blood pH! The body does an awesome job of regulating and keeping our blood at a normal pH level. To kill a myth, our bodies are not aware if we are eating a salad or a hamburger once it's gone through the digestive process. It pulls out the important nutrients the blood needs and it processes through the other organs for what they need. Healthy eating aids in achieving optimal weight, and it offers our bodies the required vitamins and nutrients it needs for long life and healthy living.

Beneficial food for health and hair growth

ALKALIZING VEGETABLES	ACIDIFYING VEGETABLES
Alfalfa	**ACIDIFYING VEGETABLES**
Barley Grass	Corn
Beet Greens	Lentils
Beets	Olives
Broccoli	Winter Squash
Cabbage	**ACIDIFYING FRUITS**
Carrot	Blueberries
Cauliflower	Canned or Glazed Fruits
Celery	Cranberries
Chard Greens	Currants

ALKALIZING VEGETABLES	ACIDIFYING VEGETABLES
Chlorella	Plums**
Collard Greens	Prunes**
Cucumber	
Dandelions	**ACIDIFYING GRAINS, GRAIN PRODUCTS**
Dulce	Amaranth
Edible Flowers	Barley
Eggplant	Bran, oat
Fermented Veggies	Bran, wheat
Garlic	Bread
Green Beans	Corn
Green Peas	Cornstarch
Kale	Crackers, soda
Kohlrabi	Flour, wheat
Lettuce	Flour, white
Mushrooms	Hemp Seed Flour
Mustard Greens	Kamut
Nightshade Veggies	Macaroni
Onions	Noodles
Parsnips (high glycemic)	Oatmeal
Peas	Oats (rolled)
Peppers	Quinoa
Pumpkin	Rice (all)
Radishes	Rice Cakes
Rutabaga	Rye
Sea Veggies	Spaghetti
Spinach, green	Spelt
Spirulina	Wheat Germ
Sprouts	Wheat
Sweet Potatoes	**ACIDIFYING BEANS & LEGUMES**
Tomatoes	Almond Milk
Watercress	Black Beans
Wheat Grass	Chick Peas
Wild Greens	Green Peas
ALKALIZING ORIENTAL VEGETABLES	Kidney Beans
Daikon	Lentils
Dandelion Root	Pinto Beans
Kombu	Red Beans
Maitake	Rice Milk

ALKALIZING VEGETABLES	ACIDIFYING VEGETABLES
Nori	Soy Beans
Rishi	Soy Milk
Shitake	White Beans
Umeboshi	**ACIDIFYING DAIRY**
Wakame	Butter
ALKALIZING FRUITS	Cheese
Apple	Cheese, Processed
Apricot	Ice Cream
Avocado	Ice Milk
Banana (high glycemic)	**ACIDIFYING NUTS & BUTTERS**
Berries	Cashews
Blackberries	Legumes
Cantaloupe	Peanut Butter
Cherries, sour	Peanuts
Coconut, fresh	Pecans
Currants	Tahini
Dates, dried	Walnuts
Figs, dried	**ACIDIFYING ANIMAL PROTEIN**
Grapes	Bacon
Grapefruit	Beef
Honeydew Melon	Carp
Lemon	Clams
Lime	Cod
Muskmelons	Corned Beef
Nectarine	Fish
Orange	Haddock
Peach	Lamb
Pear	Lobster
Pineapple	Mussels
Raisins	Organ Meats
Raspberries	Oyster
Rhubarb	Pike
Strawberries	Pork
Tangerine	Rabbit
Tomato	Salmon
Tropical Fruits	Sardines
Umeboshi Plums	Sausage
Watermelon	Scallops

ALKALIZING VEGETABLES	ACIDIFYING VEGETABLES
ALKALIZING PROTEIN	Shellfish
Almonds	Shrimp
Chestnuts	Tuna
Millet	Turkey
Tempeh (fermented)	Veal
Tofu (fermented)	Venison
Whey Protein Powder	**ACIDIFYING FATS & OILS**
ALKALIZING SWEETENERS	Avocado Oil
Stevia	Butter
ALKALIZING SPICES & SEASONINGS	Canola Oil
Chili Pepper	Corn Oil
Cinnamon	Flax Oil
Curry	Hemp Seed Oil
Ginger	Lard
Herbs (all)	Olive Oil
Miso	Safflower Oil
Mustard	Sesame Oil
Sea Salt	Sunflower Oil
Tamari	**ACIDIFYING SWEETENERS**
ALKALIZING OTHER	Carob
Alkaline Antioxidant Water	Corn Syrup
Apple Cider Vinegar	Sugar
Bee Pollen	**ACIDIFYING ALCOHOL**
Fresh Fruit Juice	Beer
Green Juices	Hard Liquor
Lecithin Granules	Spirits
Mineral Water	Wine
Molasses, blackstrap	**ACIDIFYING OTHER FOODS**
Probiotic Cultures	Catsup
Soured Dairy Products	Cocoa
Veggie Juices	Coffee
ALKALIZING MINERALS	Mustard
Calcium: pH 12	Pepper
Cesium: pH 14	Soft Drinks
Magnesium: pH 9	Vinegar
Potassium: pH 14	**ACIDIFYING DRUGS & CHEMICALS**
Sodium: pH 14	Aspirin
Although it might seem that citrus fruits would	Chemicals

ALKALIZING VEGETABLES	ACIDIFYING VEGETABLES
have an acidifying effect on the body, the citric acid they contain actually has an alkalinizing effect in the system. **Note** that a food's acid or alkaline forming tendency in the body has nothing to do with the actual pH of the food itself. For example, lemons are very acidic, however the end products they produce after digestion and assimilation are very alkaline so, lemons are alkaline forming in the body. Likewise, meat will test alkaline before digestion, but it leaves very acidic residue in the body so, like nearly all animal products, meat is very acid forming.	Drugs, Medicinal Drugs, Psychedelic Herbicides Pesticides Tobacco **ACIDIFYING JUNK FOOD** Beer: pH 2.5 Coca-Cola: pH 2 Coffee: pH 4 ** These foods leave an alkaline ash but have an acidifying effect on the body.

CHAPTER 8

Hair Care for Blood Type

Type A
Blood Type A Diet and Exercise

Type As flourish on vegetarian diets. For type A it's best to get the food source from a natural a state as possible: fresh, pure, and organic.

If you are accustomed to consuming (eating) meat, weight loss will be very rapid at first because you are eliminating toxic foods from your diet. And when you follow a Blood Type diet, your immune system becomes super charged and you short circuit potential harmful life threatening diseases from harming you.

Why it's important to eat according your Blood Type.

When Type A individuals eat meat, you may begin to experience lethargy, and sluggishness. Type A's have very low stomach acid content and with this it makes it hard to digest meat. Type A's consume little to no protein from meat and must resort to gaining protein from plants, vegetables, nuts and seeds. Protein for them is also found in beans, legumes except the foods that are on the "Do Not Eat List". Eating beans that are the "Do Not Eat List" will decrease the production of insulin in their bodies and will lead to obesity. Tofu which is high in protein and estrogen should be an essential food item in the Type A Diet.

Another type of foods that are not digested well are Dairy products. This causes the metabolism to slow down or become sluggish. By eating fermented dairy products, the Type A's digest small amounts of these dairy products.

What is of great importance to the Type A's diet are vegetables. Vegetables provide essential minerals, enzymes antioxidants and nutrients that Type A's need. They are super sensitive to an ingredient called Lectins (a type of protein found in plants) found in cabbage, peppers, potatoes- baked or sweet potatoes, tomatoes and yams (yellow). These foods aggravate the delicate lining -walls of the stomach. Eating fruits that are alkaline are best for Type A's but they should not eat manages, papaya and citrus fruits these also are not healthy for them. See the chart on page: ____________________

Vegetables are vital to the Type A's, Diet, providing minerals, enzymes and antioxidants. Type A are very sensitive to the lectins in potatoes, sweet potatoes, yams, cabbage, tomatoes and peppers. They are delicate in the stomach of Type A. Type A should eat more fruits that are alkaline, avoid mangoes, papaya and oranges for they are not good for your digestive tract.

Meat, Poultry and Seafood

Type A blood should eat plenty of fish, including salmon, sea or rainbow trout, red snapper, cod and mackerel. Chicken and poultry can be eaten up to two times a week, its best to avoid all beef, pork, game meats and shellfish.

Dairy Products and Eggs

Type A individuals may be asked to avoid all dairy products and eggs. For a substitute, try rice or soy milk. intermittently type A's might get away with eating yogurt, cream cheese, goat cheese, mozzarella cheese or kefir food without suffering any health issues.

Fruits and Vegetables

Type A individuals should eat an array of fresh, organic fruits and vegetables. The ancestors of this Blood Type A predominantly ate accordingly. By eating organic vegetable such as: artichokes, beets, onions, broccoli, okra, asparagus, cucumbers, turnips and dark leafy greens: spinach, kale, collard greens and escarole. The best suggested fruits Type A should eat are organic fruits such as blueberries, cherries, figs, avocados, pineapple, plums and grapefruit strawberries and apples.

Type A should avoid bananas, oranges, cabbage, eggplant, tomatoes and potatoes.

Grains

Sprouted wheat is an exceptional grain for type A. Cereals with buckwheat or amaranth even rice, oats, or rye flour are highly recommended in the grain family. Some grain that are not the best to eat but are acceptable Millet, rice, barely, corn couscous quinoa…suggestion is to eat only several times a week. Type A should avoid white and wheat flour & semolina pasta.

Nuts, Seeds, Beans and Legumes

Type A will benefit from lentils, black eyed peas, pumpkin seeds, peanuts, pinto beans, and legumes but they should stay away from pistachios, cashews and any type of beans naval, red, garbanzo or kidney beans.

Fats and Seasonings

Its recommended for type A to cook with and eat olive oil, canola oil or flaxseed oil. Drinking cod liver oil is beneficial. Usable seasonings include soy sauce, miso, ginger, garlic, mustard and tamari. By using self-control eating pickles, salad dressing and jams or jellies prepared from acceptable fruits are fine in moderation is fine. But completely avoid do not eat, vinegar, ketchup, mayonnaise and pepper as well as corn, peanut, sesame and safflower oils. Eating foods found in the vegan section is most beneficial. If you truly need something with a vinegary taste, try lemons and find alternative foods that does not have vinegar in it especially as a main ingredient.

Type B

For type B blood, there are two type of lectins found in foods, regular & gluten lectin. Lectins are a type of protein that attaches itself to sugars and multiply-which equals weight gain. Therefore, eating flour (bleached or whole wheat), lentils, buckwheat, sesame seeds, peanuts and or corn is not good. And these foods are loaded with this type of proteins, that effects the metabolic process which causes type B to become fatigue, sluggish and retain fluids, hypoglycemia (low blood) is potentially present. Wheat germ and whole wheat which are gluten lectin type products enhances the complications caused by other digestive-slowing foods.

Other foods that are not advisable to enjoy is sesame seeds, sunflower seeds and peanuts mainly because they interrupt the production of insulin. Consuming wheat or corn, is not tolerated either, it leads to weight gain and eating rye settles in our vascular system (blood) which causes potential strokes and blood disorders. Corn and buckwheat are major factors in Type B weight gain, they contribute to a sluggish metabolism, insulin irregularity, fluid retention, and fatigue.

Eliminate tomatoes completely (again what….) from Type B diet. It has lectins that irritate the stomach.

Type B's should consume poultry in moderation. Eating chicken which has agglutinating type lectin, (the type that sticks together and forms masses - which leads to weight gain) and the type that attacks the bloodstream potentially leading to a stroke and immune disorders. So, fish it is fish all day. Fish every day. We can eat deep ocean fish, (with mercury no thanks, guess I'll be skinny in a few months (LOL)!
One thing we can enjoy are fruits and vegetables they are generally well tolerated and should be taken liberally.

Type O
Type O Blood Type for Hair Loss

This blood is found to be overly active and hyper and at time have burst of energy at times they can concentrate on one thing. The hormones are unbalanced and weight may be an issue as well. Their responses can lead to bout of excessive temper tantrums, unexplained anger that could easily lead to a hysterical type episode. Because of how the dopamine in the blood is released they benefit with acts of rewards and positive accolades. You should encourage them more than criticize them. They are easily bored and at risk to destructive behavior when they are tired bored every sad upset.

This blood type is more likely to fall into the Trichotillomania type alopecia- this types pulls their hair out unaware at times.

The positive side here is they can be productive but with high stress levels forget about it. Their energy turns into anger, impulsive behavior even overly active behavior. Because of how they are wired with a poor diet, little to no exercise, unhealthy surroundings (environments) they are susceptible to sluggish thyroid activity, processing insulin improperly and they will even experience negative metabolic effects in the body.

This is a genetically inherited trait. It's best to purchase "iodine salt". This salt may help the thyroid to become regulated (it also helps men not to get that 'Adams Apple' in their throat). This is what leads to weight gain and retaining fluid and even exhaustion.

Do not begin to take iodine supplements unless under the strict advice of your doctor. Try considering eating foods high in salt like saltwater fish, fish that a lot of island people eat- "Salt fish", like the dish Ackee and Salt fish one of my favorite dishes…yummy.

Even can type fish (tuna, sardines, salmon) or meats (chicken, corn beef, ham). Not to eat in excess…. moderation, moderation… Believe it or not eating or becoming familiar with eating seaweed type foods is most beneficial. Eating Bladder Wrack is best for Blood Type O people. It's good for preventing hair loss and even will cause the hair to grow back. It's awesome for people trying to lose weight as well. Bladder wrack is known to improve a slow metabolic rate, according to Dr. D'Adamo.

In order, not to respond overly anxious and fall into the trap of the expected typical Type O, behavior following a restricted diet is a must!

This Type O diet would consist of:

Lean Meats	Fruits & Vegetables
Lean Chicken	Apples
Lean Beef	Grapes (except Green)
Lean Beef	Berries (blue, raspberry)
Fish	Plums
	Peaches

Eating more Alkaline foods is good. See the chart in the back of the manual for reference.

No Gluten! Eat Gluten free foods – from wheat, bread, flour, pasta, cookies, cakes.

No Caffeine or Carbonated Drinks. This stimulates and raises the adrenaline (triggers all the restlessness) For Adults no alcohol.

No Dairy Products! Avoid eggs, cheese, milk, ice cream, yogurt.

Some foods are beneficial to one blood type but harmful to another blood type. Some food will cause the digestive system to be upset.
Type O blood should undoubtedly avoid dairy products altogether. The body is not equipped to digest this type of diet. For African Americans, dairy foods such as eggs, cheese, milk, ice cream, yogurt should not be consumed.

This blood type thrives on protein from animals, not vegetable protein. Even Type O people can eat, digest and metabolize meat protein due their high stomach acids. But pay attention to the type of meat this is very important: the meat should be lean chemical free like the free-range meats, fish and poultry.

This Blood type is not like the other blood types, the diet is different and great results in lifestyle changes along with a strict diet is most beneficial.

For those wondering about weight gain, one of the leading factors in gaining weight is eating foods with gluten in it, this is one of main ingredients in wheat germ and whole wheat thus bread must be avoided, Gluten restricts the production of insulin; and slows down the metabolic rate. Also, eating beans and legumes contributes to weight gain the lectins (select protein specific for sugar a carbohydrate type protein). Another reason for weight gain is due to the low level and unstable function of the thyroid hormone. For this reason, avoid: greens including; collard, mustard, and turnip greens, cabbage, sprouts. Eating seafood, seaweeds and iodized salt is beneficial for the Type O blood person

Exercise

Persons with type O blood type are suggested to engage in exercise at least 3-4 times per week for 30-45 minutes. This blood type gets bored easily, adding variety to workouts or excising will be it fun and exciting.

To learn more about Blood Type Diet, please visit Blood Type Diet Forum or check out these books by Dr. D'Adamo called:

- Blood Type Diet O Forum - Eat Right 4 Your Blood Type O
- Blood Type Diet A Forum - Eat Right 4 Your Blood Type A
- Blood Type Diet B Forum - Eat Right 4 Your Blood Type B
- Blood Type Diet AB Forum - Eat Right 4 Your Blood Type AB

CHAPTER 9

Blood Type and Diet Connection

In my enthusiastic research regarding health and hair, I discovered Dr. Peter J. D'Adamo, ND who has done a lot of research and study on blood types and diet. While reviewing his website, history and discoveries I learned that blood type could also inadvertently and sometimes adversely impact the condition of your hair. I'd like to share with you the charts below that show how blood type and foods within certain groups can play a role in hair health.

A blood type (also called a blood group) is a classification of blood based on the presence or absence of inherited antigenic substances on the surface of red blood cells (RBCs). These antigens may be proteins, carbohydrates, glycoproteins, or glycolipids, depending on the blood group system. Some of these antigens are also present on the surface of other types of cells of various tissues.

An individual's blood type can impact overall health, including hair health with the consumption of certain foods. You can review the lists on the following pages to identify those foods that may impact your hair.
NOTE: Rxestoratives hair & skin wellness, inc® has no affiliation with Peter J. D'Adamo. There is more detailed information found on his website and in one of his many books at **http://www.dadamo.com**.

Food list description:
A = Avoid
N/B = Neutral/Beneficial
B = Beneficial
N = Neutral
- = Unknown
O = Occasional
R = Rare

DAIRY FOOD LISTS

Dairy	A	AB	B	O
Almond Milk	N	N	N	N
American Cheese	A	A	A	A
Blue Cheese	A	A	A	A
Brie Cheese	A	A	N	A
Butter	A	A	N	O
Buttermilk	A	A	N	A
Camembert Cheese	A	A	N	A
Casein	A	N	N	A
Cheddar Cheese	A	N	N	A
Colby Cheese	A	N	N	A
Cottage Cheese	A	B	B	A
Cream Cheese	A	N	N	A
Edam Cheese	A	N	N	A
Emmenthal Cheese	A	N	N	A
Farmer Cheese	N	B	B	O
Feta Cheese	N	B	B	O

Dairy	A	AB	B	O
Ghee (Clarified Butter)	N	O	O	O
Goat Cheese	N	B	B	A
Gouda Cheese	A	N	N	A
Gruyere Cheese	A	N	N	A
Half & Half	A	A	N	A
Ice Cream	A	A	A	A
Jarlsberg Cheese	A	N	N	A
Kefir	N/B	B	B	A
Milk (Cow-Skim or 2%)	R	N	B	A
Milk (Cow-Whole)	R	A	N	A
Milk (Goat)	N/B	B	B	A
Monterey Jack Cheese	A	N	N	A
Mozzarella Cheese	N/B	B	B	O
Munster Cheese	A	N	N	A
Neufchatel Cheese	A	N	N	A
Paneer	A	N	B	A
Parmesan Cheese	A	A	N	A
Provolone Cheese	A	A	N	A
Quark Cheese	A	-	N	-
Rice Milk	N	B	B	N/B
Ricotta Cheese	N/B	B	B	A

Dairy	A	AB	B	O
Sherbet	A	A	N	A
Sour Cream (low/non-fat)	N	B	N	A
Soy Cheese	B	N	N	N
Soy Milk	B	N	N	N
String Cheese	A	N	A	A
Swiss Cheese	A	N	N	A
Whey/Whey Protein Supplement	A	N	N	A
Yogurt	N	B	B	R

Food list description:
A = Avoid
N/B = Neutral/Beneficial
B = Beneficial
N = Neutral
- = Unknown
O = Occasional
R = Rare

EGG FOOD LISTS

Egg	A	AB	B	O
Duck Egg	-	-	-	-
Egg (chicken)	O?	N?	N?	O?
Egg White (chicken)	N?	B?	N?	O?
Egg Yolk (chicken)	O?	N?	N?	O?
Goose Egg	-	-	-	-
Quail Egg	-	-	-	-
Salmon Roe	-	A	A	-

Food list description:
A = Avoid
N/B = Neutral/Beneficial
B = Beneficial
N = Neutral
- = Unknown
O = Occasional
R = Rare

GRAIN FOOD LIST

Grains	A	AB	B	O
Amaranth	B	N	A	O
Artichoke Pasta (Pure)	B	A	A	O
Barley	N	N	A	O
Buckwheat/Kasha	B	A	A	N/B

Grains	A	AB	B	O
Corn	N	A	A	A
Couscous (Cracked Wheat)	N	N	A	A
Essene Bread (Manna Bread)	B	B	B	B
Ezekiel Bread	B	B	B	B
Gluten Flour	N	N	A	A
Gluten Free Bread	N	N	N	O
Graham Flour	N	N	N	A
Kamut	N	A	A	O
Millet	N	B	B	O
Oat Flour	B	B	B	an
Oat/Oat Bran/Oatmeal	N	B	B	an
Popcorn	-	-	A	A
Quinoa	N	N	N	O
Rice (Cream of)	N	N	N	N/B
Rice (Puffed)/Rice Bran	N	B	B	N/B
Rice (White/Brown/Basmati)/Bread	N	B	N	N/B
Rice (Wild)	N	B	A	O
Rice Cake/Flour	B	B	B	N/B
Rye Flour	B	B	A	O
Rye/100% Rye Bread	N	B	A	O
Soba Noodles (100% Buckwheat)	B	A	A	O
Sorghum	-	-	-	-

Grains	A	AB	B	O
Soy Flour Bread	B	B	N	N
Spelt Flour/Products	N	N	N	O
Tapioca	N	A	A	O
Teff	A	A	A	O
Wheat (Berry)	A	N	A	A
Wheat (Bleached Flour Products)	O	N	N	A
Wheat (Bran)	A	N	A	A
Wheat (Bulghur)	N	N	A	A
Wheat (Durum Flour Products)	A	N	A	A
Wheat (Germ)	A	N	A	A
Wheat (Gluten Flour Products)	N	N	A	A
Wheat (Refined UN/Bleached)	O	-	N	A
Wheat (Semolina Flour Products)	O	N	N	A
Wheat (White Flour Products)	O	N	N	A
Wheat (Whole Wheat Products)	A	N	A	A
Wheat Bread (Sprouted Commercial)	B	B	-	A

Food list description:
A = Avoid
N/B = Neutral/Beneficial
B = Beneficial
N = Neutral

- = Unknown
O = Occasional

BEAN/LENTIL FOOD LISTS

Beans/Legumes	A	AB	B	O
Adzuki Beans	B	A	A	B
Black Bean	B	A	A	O
Black Eyed Pea	B	A	A	B
Broad Bean	N	N	N	O
Cannellini Bean	N	N	N	O
Copper Bean	A	N	N	A
Fava Bean	N	A	N	O
Garbanzo Bean	A	A	A	O
Green Bean	B	N	N	O
Jicama	N	N	N	O
Kidney Bean	A	A	B	A
Lentil (Domestic)	B	N	A	A
Lentil (Green)	B	B	A	A
Lentil (Red)	B	N	A	A
Lima Bean	A	A	B	O
Mung Beans (Sprouts)	N	A	A	O
Navy Bean	A	B	B	A
Northern Bean	-	N	N	O
Pinto Bean	B	B	A	B
Red Bean	A	B	N	O

Beans/Legumes	A	AB	B	O
Snap Bean	N	N	N	O
Soy Bean	B	B	B	O
Soy Flakes	-	N	-	-
Soy Granules	-	N	-	-
Tamarind Bean	A	N	N	A
Tempeh (Fermented Soy)	B	B	A	O
Tofu	B	B	A	O
White Bean	N	N	N	O

Food list description:
A = Avoid
N/B = Neutral/Beneficial
B = Beneficial
N = Neutral
- = Unknown
O = Occasional
R = Rare

VEGETABLE FOOD LISTS

Vegetable/Veg Juice	A	AB	B	O
Acacia (Arabic Gum)	A	A	A	A
Agar	N	N	N	N
Alfalfa Sprouts	B	B	N	A
Aloe/Aloe Tea/Aloe Juice	B	A	A	A

Vegetable/Veg Juice	A	AB	B	O
Artichoke	B	A	A	B
Arugula	N	N	N	N
Asparagus	N	N	N	N
Bamboo Shoot	N	N	N	N
Beet	N	B	B	N
Beet Greens	B	B	B	B
Beet/Beet Greens Juice	N	B	B	N
Bok Choy	N	N	N	N
Broccoli	B	B	B	B
Brussel Sprout	N	N	B	A
Cabbage (Chinese/Red/White)	A	N	B	A
Cabbage Juice	N	B	B	A
Caper	A	A	N	A
Carrot	B	N	B	N
Carrot Juice	B	B	N	N
Cauliflower	N	B	B	A
Celeriac	-	-	-	-
Celery	N	B	N	N
Celery Juice	B	B	N	N
Chervil	N	N	N	N
Chicory	B	N	N	B
Cilantro	N	-	-	-
Collard Greens	B	B	B	B

Vegetable/Veg Juice	A	AB	B	O
Cucumber	N	B	N	N
Cucumber Juice	N	N	N	N
Daikon Radish	N	N	N	N
Eggplant	A	B	B	A
Endive	N	N	N	N
Escarole	B	N	N	B
Fennel	N	N	N	N
Fiddlehead Fern	N	N	N	N
Garlic	B	B	N	B
Ginger	B	N	B	N
Horseradish	B	N	N	B
Kale	B	B	B	B
Kelp	N	N	N	B
Kohlrabi	B	N	N	B
Leek	B	N	N	B
Lettuce	N	N	N	N
Lettuce (Romaine)	B	N	N	B
Mushroom (Abalone)	N	A	N	N
Mushroom (Domestic)	A	N	N	A
Mushroom (Oyster/Enoki/Portobello)	N	N	N	N
Mushroom (Shiitake)	A	A	B	A
Mushroom (Straw)	N	-	-	-
Mustard Greens	N	B	B	A

Vegetable/Veg Juice	A	AB	B	O
Okra	B	N	N	B
Olive (Black)	A	A	A	A
Olive (Greek/Spanish)	A	N	A	A
Onion (Green)	N	N	N	N
Onion (Red/Spanish/Yellow)	B	N	N	B
Parsnip	B	B	B	B
Pea (Green/Pod/Snow)	N	N	N	N
Pepper (Green/Yellow/Jalapeno)	A	A	B	N
Pepper (Red/Cayenne)	A	A	B	B
Pickle	N	A	N	A
Pimento	N	N	N	N
Potato (Sweet)	A	B	B	B
Potato (White/Red/ Blue/Yellow)	A	N	N	A
Pumpkin	B	N	A	B
Radicchio	N	N	N	N
Radish	N	A	A	N
Radish Sprouts	N	A	A	N
Rappini	N	N	N	N
Rhubarb	A	A	A	A
Rutabaga	N	N	N	N

Vegetable/Veg Juice	A	AB	B	O
Sauerkraut	A	N	-	A
Scallion	N	N	N	N
Shallots	N	N	N	N
Spinach/Spinach Juice	B	N	N	B
Spirulina/Spirulina Juice	-	-	-	A
Squash (Summer/Winter)	N	N	N	N
String Bean	N	N	N	N
Swiss Chard	B	N	N	B
Taro	N	-	-	-
Tomato/Tomato Juice	A	N	A	N
Turnip	B	N	N	B
Water Chestnut	N	N	N	N
Watercress	N	N	N	N
Yam	A	B	B	N
Yucca	-	-	-	N
Zucchini	N	N	N	N

Food list description:
A = Avoid
N/B = Neutral/Beneficial
B = Beneficial
N = Neutral
- = Unknown
O = Occasional
R = Rare

PROTEIN FOOD LISTS

Meat	A	AB	B	O
Bacon/Ham/Pork	Avoid	Avoid	Avoid	Avoid
Beef	A	A	Neutral	Beneficial
Buffalo	A	A	N	B
Chicken	O	A	A	N
Cornish Hens	O	A	A	N
Duck	A	A	A	N
Goat	A	A	-	N
Goose	A	A	A	A
Heart	A	A	A	B
Lamb	A	B	B	B
Liver (Calf)	A	O	N	B
Mutton	A	B	B	B
Partridge	R	A	A	N
Pheasant	A	O	O	N
Quail	R	A	A	N
Rabbit	A	B	B	N
Turkey	O	B	O	N/B
Turtle	A	A	A	N
Veal	A	A	N	B
Venison	A	A	B	B

Food list description:
A = Avoid
N/B = Neutral/Beneficial
B = Beneficial
N = Neutral
- = Unknown
O = Occasional
R = Rare

FISH FOOD LISTS

Fish	A	AB	B	O
Abalone	N	N	N	N
Anchovy	A	A	A	N
Barracuda	A	A	A	A
Bass (Bluegill)	A	A	A	N
Bass (Sea)	N	A	A	N
Bass (Striped)	A	A	A	B
Beluga	A	A	A	N
Bluefish	A	N	N	B
Carp	B	N	N	N
Catfish	A	N	N	A
Caviar	A	N	B	A
Clam	A	A	A	N
Cod	B	B	B	B
Conch	A	A	A	A
Crab	A	A	A	N
Crab (Horseshoe)	-	A	A	-
Crayfish/Crawfish	A	A	A	N

Fish	A	AB	B	O
Eel/Japanese Eel	A	A	A	N
Flounder	A	A	B	N
Frog	A	A	A	N
Gray Sole	A	A	-	N
Grouper	A	B	B	N
Haddock	A	A	B	N
Hake	A	A	B	B
Halibut	A	A	B	B
Herring/Kippers (fresh)	A	N	N	B
Herring/Kippers (pickled)	A	A	N	A
Lobster	A	A	A	N
Lox	A	A	A	A
Mackerel	B	B	B	B
Mahi mahi	N	B	B	N
Monkfish	B	B	B	N/B
Mussels	A	N	A	N
Octopus	A	A	A	A
Oyster	A	A	A	N
Perch (Ocean)	N	B	B	N
Perch (Silver)	B	N	N	N
Perch (White)	N	N	N	B
Perch (Yellow)	B	N	N	B
Pickerel	B	B	B	N

Fish	A	AB	B	O
Pike	N	B	B	B
Sailfish	N	B	N	N
Salmon (Ocean: Pacific NW, Norwegian)	B	N	B	B
Salmon (Farm Raised)	N	N	N	N
Sardine	B	B	B	B
Scallop	A	N	N	N
Shad	A	B	B	B
Shark	N	N	N	N
Shrimp	A	A	A	N
Smelt	N	N	N	N/B
Snail (Helix Pomatia/Escargot)	B	B	A	N
Snapper	N	N	N	B
Sole	A	A	B	B
Squid	A	N	N	N
Sturgeon	N	B	B	B
Swordfish	N	N	N	B
Tilefish	A	N	N	B
Trout (Rain/Bow)	B	B	N	B
Trout (Sea)	B	B	B	N
Tuna	N	B	N	N/B
Weakfish	N	N	N	N
Whitefish	B	N	N	B

Fish	A	AB	B	O
Yellowtail	N	A	A	B

Food list description:
A = Avoid
N/B = Neutral/Beneficial
B = Beneficial
N = Neutral
- = Unknown
O = Occasional
R = Rare

JUICE FOOD LISTS

Fruit/Fruit Juice	A	AB	B	O
Apple	N	N	N	N
Apple Cider/Apple Juice	N	N	N	A
Apricot/Apricot Juice	B	N	N	N
Avocado	N	A	A	A
Banana	A	A	B	N/B
Blackberry/Blackberry Juice	B	N	N	A
Blueberry	B	N	N	N/B
Boysenberry	B	N	N	N
Canang Melon	N	N	N	N
Cantaloupe	A	N	N	A
Casaba Melon	N	N	N	N
Cherry (Bing, Sweet, White, etc)	B	B	N	N

Fruit/Fruit Juice	A	AB	B	O
Cherry/Juice (Black)	B	B	N	B
Christmas Melon	N	N	N	N
Coconut/Coconut Milk	A	A	A	A
Cran/Berry	B	B	B	N
Cran/Berry Juice	N	B	B	N
Crenshaw Melon	N	N	N	N
Currants (Black/Red)	N	N	N	N
Date	N	N	N	N
Elderberry (Dark Blue/Purple)	N	N	N	N
Fig (Fresh/Dried)	B	B	N	B
Gooseberry	N	B	N	N
Grape	N	B	B	N
Grapefruit	B	B	N	N
Grapefruit Juice	B	N	N	N
Guava	N	A	N	N/B
Guava Juice	N	-	-	-
Honeydew	A	N	N	A
Jam/Jelly OK'd Ingred	N	N	N	N
Kiwi	N	B	N	N
Kumquat	N	N	N	N

Fruit/Fruit Juice	A	AB	B	O
Lemon/Lemon Juice	B	B	N	N
Lime/Lime Juice	N	N	N	N
Logan Berry	N	B	N	N
Mango/Mango Juice	A	A	N	N/B
Musk Melon	N	N	N	N
Nectarine/Nectarine Juice	N	N	N	N
Orange/Orange Juice	A	A	N	A
Papaya	A	N	B	N
Papaya Juice	A	B	B	N
Peach	N	N	N	N
Pear/Pear Juice	N	N	N	N
Persimmon	N	A	A	N
Pineapple	B	B	B	N
Pineapple Juice	B	N	B	B
Plantain	A	N	N	A
Plum (Dark/Green/Red)	B	B	B	B
Pomegranate	N	A	A	N
Prickly Pear	N	A	A	N
Prune/Prune Juice	B	N	N	B
Raisin	B	N	N	N

Fruit/Fruit Juice	A	AB	B	O
Raspberry	N	N	N	N
Spanish Melon	N	N	N	N
Starfruit (Carambola)	N	A	A	N
Strawberry	N	N	N	A
Tangerine/ Tangerine Juice	A	N	N	A
Water & Lemon	B	N	N	-
Watermelon	N	N	N	N
Tangerine/ Tangerine Juice	A	N	N	A

CHAPTER 10

Herbs for Hair Growth

Son 4:13 You are an orchard that puts forth pomegranates and other precious fruits, henna and nard —
Son 4:14 nard, saffron and aromatic cane, cinnamon and all kinds of frankincense trees, myrrh, aloes, all the best spices.
Son 4:15 You are a garden fountain, a spring of running water, flowing down from the L'vanon. CJB

I have complied a list of known, tried and tested ingredients for Hair Growth. You will find 33 herbs that are great for hair growth.

33+ Best Herbs for Hair Growth

Aloe Vera or enzymes in Aloe Vera causes the dead skin cells to disband and sebum in excess can clog hair follicles. This herb naturally contains salicylic acid which is an anti-inflammatory and is a light antibiotic. The gel in Aloe Vera acts as an excellent moisturizer which is similar to keratin an awesome protein beneficial for skin and hair. As an herb this herb is the best carrier for other herbs and herbal remedies. This herb is best for promoting hair growth. Aloe Vera may spoil a formula if the right preservative is not added to the mixture.

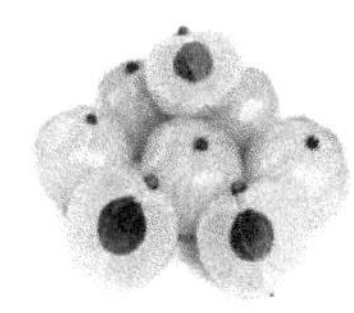

Amla herbs contain several antioxidants including the best one known to the average consumer Vitamin C. Amla known as an Indian Gooseberry is necessary for collagen production when combined with this Vitamin. Higher levels of collagen accelerate the production and increase strength for new hair growth. Note: Amla is also an excellent remedy for premature graying of hair.

Basil is a stimulant and known to promote hair growth. This herb is rich in magnesium and is an essential mineral when processed in the body. As an herbal rinse, basil becomes an anti-flammatory which strengthens the hair against breakage. When massaged into the scalp, this herb improves circulation and promotes hair growth along with healing and results in a healthy scalp. When blended with burdock root, fenugreek and lavender, the herb offers supreme healing attributes.

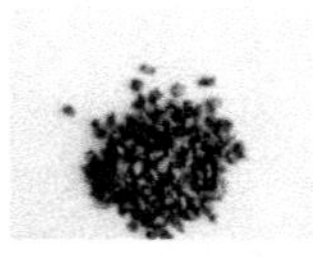

Burdock Root Herb is anti-inflammatory rich in fatty acids. Burdock root oil can be used alone or combined with other herbs such as rosemary, lavender, or sage to improve scalp health and stimulate new hair growth.

Calendula flowers or Oil is very popular and known as the marigold flower. It is rich in minerals and anti-oxidants. This plant is known in the herbal community as Calendula, when applied to the scalp the hairs grows back stronger and healthier the collagen production is increased and blood circulation is increased where the follicles are concerned. This herb/flower can be combined with other moisturizing oils or herbs.

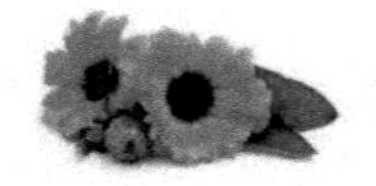

Carrot Root that becomes an oil is superb in regenerating and stimulating the follicle and skin cells. It is very high carotenes and other antioxidants. This oil contains Retin-A this a form of vitamin A it used with Rogaine in a synthetic form to support hair growth in men with male pattern baldness. For people who are experiencing hair loss need to invest in this oil or products with this oil in its purest form in NOT synthetic form.

Carrot Seed is good if you need detoxing the body using the herb is phenomenal, but for uses in hair care and skin it's great for stimulating hair follicles and relieving the skin from being dull dry ashy and itchy. It is known as for its nice aroma too.

Cedarwood Oil works at times bacterial infections cause hair loss and hinders hair growth. The immune system is at times suffers from deficiencies from the diet. This oil/herb used alone will combat this issue its best for people who suffer with alopecia.

Chamomile, German is good at times there is inflammation of the scalp which includes the hair follicles where hair loss soon follows. Chamomile known as an effective inflammation reducer to use on the scalp offer great results. Chamomile is known to soothe and cool down areas that's over heated. The fragrance of this herb is nice especially when mixed with lavender which has the same effect.

Clary Sage is the only herb to balance hormones in men and women, as it pertains to hair growth. It balances estrogen hormone levels in women but is vital when dealing with healthy skin and hair producing scalp. this herb is great for the mature women experiencing hair loos especially if it is due menopause.

Clove has definite stimulation for hair growth for a natural powerful antiseptic and for creating circulation of the scalp and follicles for hair growth, this herb fresh or in oil form is one the most power potent antioxidant naturally. When mixed with other stimulating herbs you have a great product to regrow hair. This herb is great for painful tooth aches as well. Do your research on this we are talking about hair ☺

Coltsfoot- This beautiful bright yellow flower is known in the herbal community to relieve congestion and other respiratory problems. When used as an infusion or tincture drinking with honey this is a great natural alternative. Speaking of respiratory problems with regular consumption the leaves aids in asthma, colds and hacking coughs even sinus problems. Known to be an anti-inflammatory, the antioxidant properties are promising as well. This herb or oil helps alleviate microbial functions making the skin to look younger with use. When combined with Horsetail and Neetle this herb stimulates hair growth at a rapid speed.

Cypress has the benefits of the herbs is phenomenal it has the most amazing ability to increase circulation and to strengthen capillaries. With good blood circulation, the follicle can grow. Different formulas include cypress and add Gingko to optimum blood circulation that deals specifically with the scalp.

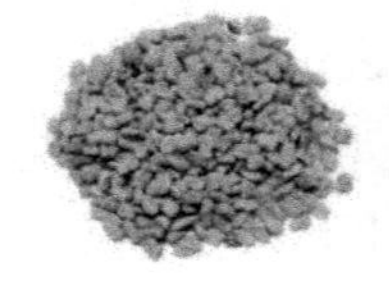

Fenugreek is a sweet-smelling fenugreek is a plant with an ancient background as both culinary seasoning and natural remedy. Fenugreek rich in vitamins and minerals this herb is known to improve circulation and it also is a stimulant meaning it stimulate hair growth especially when applied as a paste on the scalp for 30 minutes or more....see the formula in chapter 14.

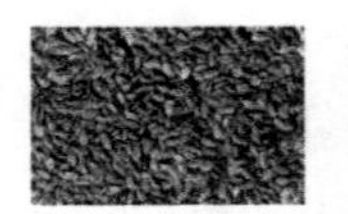

Flaxseed or the seeds of the flax plant are well-known for their **dietary health benefits** on the mind and body. Also, known as linseed. Full of fatty acids and antioxidants, ground flax seeds boiled in water will form a soothing gel that can be applied to scalp and hair to moisturize skin, eliminate dandruff, stimulate new growth, and improve the strength of existing hair. For a guide on making flax seed gel, check out this **article**. Flax oil can also be taken as a **supplement** or try adding **ground flaxseed** to food to improve scalp health and circulation, among a long list of other benefits.

Ginger Root increases circulation concerning hair follicles. This root encourages strong healthy hair that enables hair to grow faster. Not only does it make the hair grow faster but it is also an antiseptic and moisturizer, which makes it an excellent cleanser for clearing up dandruff and other skin conditions which could interfere with healthy hair growth.

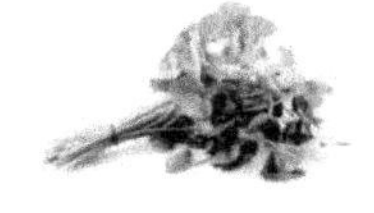

Gotu Kola, also known as Brahmi, is an ancient herb used in traditional medicine to treat a wide variety of internal and external maladies. Gotu kola extract added to olive oil can be massaged into the scalp to improve circulation and encourage new hair growth.

Helichrysum/Helichrysum is for mature skin and healing wounds even scar tissue. Helichrysum is known to regenerate soft tissue and heal scar tissue in the body. It's an excellent anti-inflammatory and it enhances circulation. It is considered to act the same for the scalp as well. Some doctors when dealing with older people would consider this herb to be beneficial for regenerating skin for the elderly scalp because it resembles scar tissue.

Horsetail Herb is naturally enriched with silica or silicon, this mineral alone strengthens our bones, nails and hair. It assists in not only making the hair strong but allows for high sheen and will improve the texture of the hair as well. Another mineral that is prevalent in this herb is selenium this is the ingredient that grows the hair and helps to make each strand follicle strong. Selenium helps the body process iodine, and this regulates hair growth also. If there is a deficiency in this mineral hair loss will

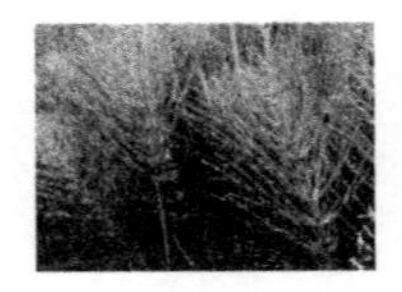

follow. Ingesting horsetail whether in tea food, or topical it needed in the body for bones, strong long healthy hair, beautiful nails.

Hibiscus flowers contain vitamins and antioxidants that improves the health of the scalp and hair. Using fresh or dried blossoms is most beneficial for hair growth. And a plus is its said to help decrease gray hair and dandruff.

When applied to scalp and hair regularly, this mixture increases hair growth while at the same time warding off premature graying and dandruff. For best results, allow mixture to soak into scalp and hair for at least two hours.
Hibiscus flowers – either fresh or dried – can be added to coconut oil and ground into a fine paste. When applied to scalp and hair regularly, this mixture works to reverse hair loss, as well as to prevent premature graying and reduce dandruff. This treatment works best if allowed to soak into scalp and hair for two hours or more.

[10] Hops flowers are widely recognized for their ability to stimulate hair growth as well as to strengthen existing hair and reduce breakage. Hops flower oil is also a natural antiseptic which can help to prevent hair loss caused by microbial infection of the hair and scalp follicles.
Horsetail is rich in minerals and extremely popular for promoting a healthy scalp and hair growth, works by stimulating blood vessels that supply oxygen to the hair follicles. Horsetail has antiviral and anti-allergy abilities. It contains silica which assist in repairing damaged hair and it fortify new and existing hair against breakage. It contains collagen

---

[10] www.healthyplants.wsu.us

minerals calcium and is an antioxidant.

Irish Moss straight from the Atlantic Ocean this seaweed is full of nutrients it has binding (emulsifying) benefits. This herb offers a youthful characteristic to it. Beneficial for hair nails and skin. Some of the minerals found in Irish Moss is beta carotene, iodine, potassium, amino acids, Vitamins A, B, C, D, E, F and K the most important that our hair and skin needs is sulfur. This herb will combine with other oils, liquids it acts as a stabilizer. When this herb is submerged in hot water (boiling the water at first) it produces mucilage, a gooey, gummy like feel to it.

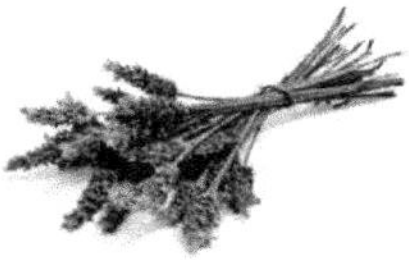

Lavender is known as a soothing, anti-bacterial, regenerative and an anti-flammatory, and an antiseptic herb. This herb is great for all hair types and any type of scalp condition. It is used to relieve stress and to prevent dry hair/scalp. as a stimulant, its great the scalp. Lavender strengthens hair from the root and helps to balance sebum on the scalp. Lavender oil is an excellent insect repellent. It even wards of disease carrying insects like fleas, head lice, mosquitos, even ticks. It blends well with other essential oils.

Licorice root contains several chemical compounds that has the ability to reverse chemical damage of the hair and scalp. it can prevent hair loss, treat dandruff, heal fungus infection the flavonoids naturally occur in licorice root. Its beneficial to nourish the scalp and heal eczema and its known to be a cleanser as well.

Marshmallow or the roots of Marshmallow have lauric acid and is found in the medium fatty acids the same found in coconut oil which is the reason its full of health benefits. This root is rich in mucilage which is known to be a naturally detangle hair. See the treatment section for the formula.

Myrtle will balance over producing sebum in the scalp and help to unclog

the pores and follicles. This herb is a natural antiseptic that is gentle and considered to be regenerative herb.
. Use at.5 - 1%.

Oat straw herb is another herbal source of silica and magnesium they both promote healthy scalps and healthy hair. An herbal rinse used with this herb- regrowing hair is promising. For prolong hair growth consider drinking this herb as well.

Parsley is easy to grow in most climates, Petroselinium crispum – common garden parsley is full of vitamins and antioxidants which increase keratin and collagen production in the scalp, increase circulation, promote healthy hair growth, and protect skin and hair from damage by free radicals. Parsley also contains zinc and copper which work together to regulate metabolism and synthesize melanin, the pigment that protects skin and hair from sun damage. Create an herbal rinse by steeping parsley in boiling water or grind fresh parsley mixed with water or oil into a fine paste to be applied to scalp and hair. Parsley can also be added to tea and salads; however pregnant women should avoid ingesting large amounts of parsley as the herb can potentially cause miscarriage.

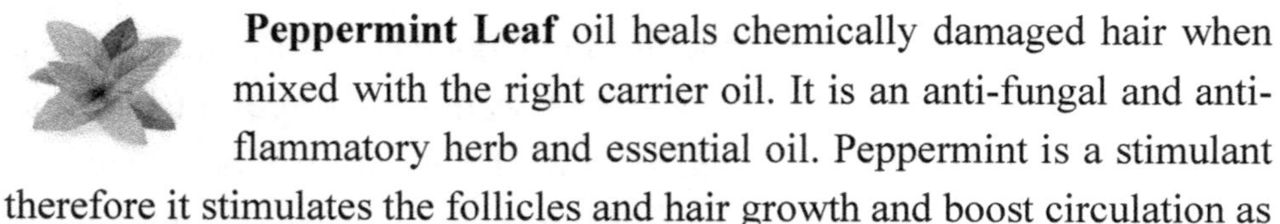

Peppermint Leaf oil heals chemically damaged hair when mixed with the right carrier oil. It is an anti-fungal and anti-flammatory herb and essential oil. Peppermint is a stimulant therefore it stimulates the follicles and hair growth and boost circulation as well. This is known to be a moisturizing oil also.

Rose Hips is considered a fruit, rose hips is the best source of Vitamin C the same amount found in oranges. This fruit which is dried into an herb is a stimulant that good for hair growth. See the formula in the treatment section

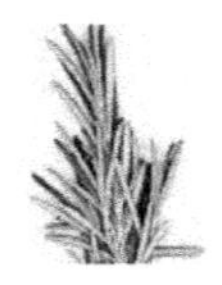

Rosemary grows in just about any type of climate. Rosemary

essential oil is rich in vitamins. It is also anti-bacterial, antioxidant, and is very effective in hair growth. This oil can be used alone, added to a scalp treatment or conditioner you may have already. Highly regarded for hair growth, with stimulating properties found in Rosemary along with hormone balancing of Clary Sage. Can balance scalp oils, and is found in blends for scar reduction and skin regeneration.[11]

[12] **Sage** is another herb widely used in the hair care industry. Sage essential oil (EO) is beneficial for controlling dandruff and treating hair loss. It is medically beneficial because of its high vitamin nutrient value of B, A and C including the minerals of potassium and calcium. This EO is not for children or if pregnant. Use at.5 - 1%. Sage is credited with many healing qualities, its known to be a calming herb. This valued herb contains vitamins which improve the growth and strength of hair, it has vitamins B and C, magnesium, zinc, and potassium. Sage has antibiotic and anti-allergic, and antiseptic properties making it ideal for healing skin ailments that may stunt hair growth. Add sage oil to a moisturizer or create an herbal rinse by steeping dried sage in hot water. A stimulating herb for hair growth is highly recommended-when used with Clary Sage its known to be a hormone balancer when taken as tea. This herb (fresh, dried or EO) can reduce skin irritations and the appearance of scars. This herb is prevalently used throughout hair care products for its beneficial properties. Its known to control even managed dandruff. It is also high in vitamins A, B & C plus is full of important mineral such as calcium and potassium. This EO is not for children or if pregnant. Use at.5 - 1%. [13]

Sea Buckthorn has been noted as enhancing skin and scalp health for

---

[11] Ulrike Blume-Peytavi, author of “Hair Growth and Disorders.”

[12] www,plantsystems

[13] Ulrike Blume-Peytavi, author of “Hair Growth and Disorders.”

every skin type and even every imbalance. Highly nutritive, potent antioxidant and regenerative. Due to high carotene content, will tend to leave the scalp with a little red color for a while after applied - be careful not to stain clothes and bedding. May prevent UV damage, which has been implicated in reducing energy in hair follicles. This is an amazing oil, well worth its berry-redness! Noted as enhancing skin and scalp health for every skin type and even every imbalance. Highly nutritive, potent antioxidant and regenerative. Use at.5 2%.

Stinging Nettle has been observed in some studies to relieve symptoms of BPH, it is a belief without concrete proof that this herb can inhibit the conversion of testosterone to follicle-harming dihydrotestosterone (DHT). Remember there are no clinical studies that have been conducted to this date on its ability to combat hair loss and its mechanism of action in regards to treating BPH remains unknown, all nettle root extract is a popular ingredient in herbal and natural, hair loss treatments along with the other assumed DHT blockers such as saw palmetto.
This herb does not actually sting but it is known to stimulate hair growth while prohibiting the production of DHT. Combine with Horsetail and Colts foot for an excellent hair and scalp treatment

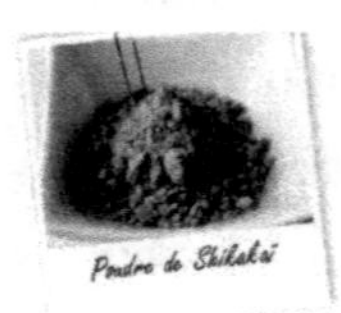

Shikakai is another naturally grown soap/cleanser herb, found in Asia it is use as a Hair cleanser as well. Best when used as a dried herb it can be easily ground up into a power or steeped in water to make a liquid cleanser. To promote hair growth, make a paste into a powder to improved the scalp follicles and strengthen the hair. This herb when turned into a powder combined with alma is an excellent antioxidant and anti-microbial most beneficial for dark colored hair.

Soapnut or the fruit of Soapnut, we know it as Lychee, in many countries they this for soap it's a natural cleanser with anti-inflammatory and anti-microbial properties allows this herb. This fruit is not edible but most useful in the household chores. Formula found in back of the book

Tea Tree EO is a very powerful immune stimulant. This EO helps to fight three (3) infectious organisms (bacteria, fungi, and viruses), it helps by destroying it at the root. It's also beneficial in fighting against acne of the skin, dandruff even lice. Its Anti-microbial means it destroys microbes, antiviral it helps by rupturing cyst in colds viruses, anti-bacterial EO.

Thyme is full of minerals magnesium potassium and selenium these minerals and vitamins promote hair growth. It is known to have antiseptic and anti-fungal properties, adding this herb to the list of treatments for damaging scalp ailments. This herbs promotes stronger hair from the root, follicles to the ends. When used as a dried herb a warm water an herbal rinse of Thyme is very advantageous its best categorize this with damaged hair and aging scalps.

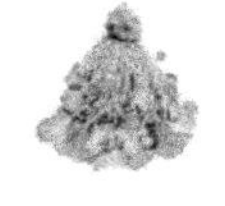

Watercress is rich in minerals and vitamins loaded with biotin naturally this herb makes the hair and skin healthier and stronger. Watercress as a rinse is out-of-this-world for hair growth.

Yarrow is anti-inflammatory, antiseptic, and astringent herb making it an ideal remedy for treating scalp conditions which can cause hair loss. Add a few drops of yarrow oil to a carrier oil such as jojoba or olive to help stimulate new hair growth.

Yucca is not the vegetable that islanders enjoy eating this is a succulent plant that has natural nourishing and cleansing effects on the scalp and hair. This plant is excellent for use in shampoo and soaps.

Ylang Ylang like Lavender, it is thought to reduce stress. Long used to increase the thickness of the hair shaft and to grow thicker hair. Can have a balancing effect on scalp oil production, and may help with split ends. Use.5 - 1%[14]

Watercress is an antioxidant, a key ingredient for the prevention of cancer. Antioxidants prevent cells from being damaged and stop free radicals from running wildly throughout our bodies as for hair care it is richly packed with vitamins and minerals including zinc, iron, and biotin – all of which have proven benefits for scalp and hair health. For a healthy metabolism use this as a tea with natural sweeteners. Being loaded with potassium this acts as a natural diuretic that draws out water from the body.

Xanthum Gum thickener is needed for all Rinses to make less watery, runny.

NOTE: The above herbs are available for purchase thru Rxestoratives H&S Wellness® Finally, there is a wide array of EOs that contain nutrients which may help to prevent and reverse hair loss.

---

[14] http://www.anandaapothecary.com/articles/hair-growth-essential-oils.html

CHAPTER 11

Oils for Hair Growth

Exo. 25:6 Oil for the light, spices for anointing oil, and for sweet incense, KJV
Exo. 30:25 And thou shalt make it an oil of holy ointment, an ointment compound after the art of the apothecary: it shall be an holy anointing oil.

What do Hair Oils Do?

Every carrier oil and EO has its specific use. The most widely used base or carrier oils for hair care is Jojoba oil (this is a wax) and Coconut oil. Grapeseed oil is good for the skin and nails. These oils are also used to moisturize the hair and protect it from the damaging rays of the sun. Essential oils (EO) feed the hair and protect it and can help treat the scalp if there are skin problems.

As explained before, there is an EO available for nearly every hair or scalp problem. These oils are easy to get hold of in vitamin shops or health food stores and often have more than one use; EOs can also be added to a bath (only a few drops will do). You need to be sure when buying hair oils as you may not clearly understand what type of oil you need or that is beneficial for your hair

Oils & Butters for Hair Growth, Shine and Strengthening

Carrier Oils and Butters benefit for Hair are listed below.

Carrier oils is defined as such because they "carry" an essential oil (EO) to the skin. Carrier oils refer to base oils that are used to dilute EOs before applying them directly to your skin. You'll find each carrier oil has different properties which may benefit one person more than another for various reasons. Each Carrier oil performs different when used for specific reasons.

Remember to always label blended carrier oils and EOs, it is best to store carrier oils and EO in glass bottles. This helps to preserve them longer. Carrier oils are typically cold-pressed oils that are produced from the fatty portions of a specific plant. Carrier oils do not evaporate like Essential Oils (EO's) do, and carrier oils can go rancid where (EO's) will not, especially when a preservative has not been added to it.

The main carrier oils are listed below: Typically, most oils purchased at a grocery store will not be cold-pressed, with the exception of olive oil and a few others (read the label first). Oils that are not cold-pressed have been heated and have a minimal therapeutic effect. The color is the give-away. So, when you purchase a carrier oil listed below, make sure they are natural. Health food stores are probably your best bet. The only exception I would make is an oil that has natural Vitamin E (like Wheat Germ Oil) because it acts as natural preservative.
What about Mineral oil? Mineral oil is not used in aromatherapy because mineral oil does not penetrate the skin, it will clog the skin and if you are having skin irritations this ingredient will burn the skin or even irritate more. Since mineral oil cannot be absorbed the EO will not be absorbed either. For this specific reason, I do not recommend replacing mineral oil with any other carrier oil, especially when making castor oil products.

Almond Oil, Sweet
Almond Oil or Sweet almond oil act as a "sealant." Almond Oil locks in" moisture. Sweet almond oil nourishes hair, smooth hair cuticles which leads to stopping /preventing shedding. This Carrier Oil promotes hair growth and thickness, prevents hair loss, and elevates shine to a natural new level.

Hair with proper nourishment, daily or weekly scalp massages prevents hair loss by incorporating Sweet Almond Oil this leads to stronger hair over time with a which is most beneficial to hair growth.

Argan oil
This carrier oil is new to the 'carrier oil' phenome…. It is the most expensive of the carrier oils. It contains an array of vitamin E, Omega 3 and 9 fatty acids, and antioxidants, all of which do amazing things for damaged, dry, coarse or otherwise unmanageable hair.

There are several smoothing products on the market containing Argan oil, but you'll get the best results applying it using the method at the top of this list. This carrier oil can be used by itself with great healing results

Avocado Oil Butter

Avocado oil contains proteins, healthy fats, amino acids and vitamins A, D, E and B6. The proteins will help fill in damaged done to the hair's cuticles also will aid in repairing damaged tresses that will prevent future breakage and frizz. Avocado oil is strong and thick, so it is most effective when used on medium to thick hair. By adding the proper EO makes for a phenomenal restorative treatment. This oil is similar to Argan oil

Beeswax

Comes from the honeycomb it is anti-microbial and used as an emollient. This is a wax that offers a film to protect the skin against pollution and this wax allows the skin to breathe unlike petrochemicals. It is high in vitamin A which makes it anti-inflammatory and anti-bacterial and even non-allergenic. This wax locks in moisture so using it in hair and skin products is beneficial.

Borage Oil

To slow down or decrease the aging process and harm caused by UV rays this oil is used to decrease inflammatory swelling like under eye bags.

Broccoli Oil

To have healthy hair we need important vitamins and broccoli has vitamin A, C and calcium. Broccoli is considered a dark green leafy vegetable which makes it of most importance to the hair. This is considered a superfood for internal hair care and with the use of the oil its beneficial for external care as well.

Broccoli promotes hair growth by stimulating and producing sebum this acts as natural moisturizer/conditioner for the scalp and hair the calcium that is in this oil strengthens the hair follicles.

Castor Oil

For both dry hair and a dry scalp, castor oil provides an effective solution. Massaged into the hair will strengthen it and eliminate dandruff, lice, fleas, and other scalp problems. Will also thicken thin hair and eyebrows. Mixed with Coconut Oil, it will blacken hair and mixed with cocoa butter, it will make it grow, & tone skin color.

Castor oil is considered a rich fatty acid is soothing and lubricating. It is a carrier oil that attracts moisture to the hair and skin. It is commonly used in hair products such as hair oils, balms and other thick emulsions for the skin and hair. When used in combinations with other oils especially EO a phenomenal hair treatments are created. Great for chemically treated damaged hair, dry dull hair, hot oil treatments, over processed hair. See EO chart on pages 146-148.

Omega 9 fatty acids found in castor oil, act as a great moisturizer, thereby helping to prevent scalp dryness. Using castor oil on a regular basis is the simplest way to ensure regrowth of hair. Those complaining about thinning of hair can use castor oil, as it assists to thicken hair.

Coco Butter
As a natural fat extractor and as a natural butter it comes from seeds by roasting them from the tropical cocoa tree. This butter is hard to the touch but will melt at body temperature. It is an emollient and will soften the skin when applied with other ingredients. It is highly moisturizing and most beneficial for hair treatments.

Coconut Oil
Another oil that has been effective to encourage hair growth is coconut oil when it comes to proper hair care. It is inexpensive and considered to be a very good option for conditioning the hair. This carrier oil is high in vitamin E and other nutrients; it's one of the most powerful oils in the world. It contains anti-microbial properties and has beneficial acids such as lauric and capric acid. By it having amazing anti-microbial powers this means it will make your hair and scalp healthier and prevent dandruff, itchy scalp and infections. These types of acids are known to prevent dandruff and itchy scalps. It's high in several other vitamins and nutrients as well. As vitamins and minerals do make up an important part of the ingredients of Coconut Oil, when applied to the scalp it not only improves hair growth but also helps to correct damaged hair. For the clients' hair, the results will be thicker, shiner, healthier and stronger hair and roots. This is all most beneficial for the hair.
Coconut oils are used in hair creams and balms and EO can be used either warm or cold. Applied to the hair and left on for at least an hour (cover hair with plastic) it moisturizes the hair and calms the scalp. This is especially beneficial after hair dye, chemical treatments or after being in the sun all day.

This oil can be combined with other nice smelling EOs that are great for hair and skin. Coconut Oil & Grape seed Oil are especially beneficial for dry hair suffering from indoor heating and sun. The hair is nourished and will regain its elasticity after a treatment with this oil. Apply the oil to towel dry hair; leave on for half an hour. Great for at home treatment, treat hair with heat for 15 to 20 minutes for best results.

Note: Make sure to purchase Extra Virgin Coconut Oil. This will allow for maximum effectiveness – Available from Rxestoratives Coconut Oil.

Grapeseed Oil

Grapeseed oil should be used as a hot oil treatment for best results. This oil has many benefits: it offers great sheen, it reduces brittleness, relieves dandruff, flakey scalps. Its known by naturopaths to solve/reduce the problem of seborrheic dermatitis. This oil contains Vitamin & Linoleic Acid these two ingredients makes the follicles healthy and stronger. The cuticles of each strand are smoother moistures is sealed in after the use of Grapeseed oil. This oil is great for those who use flat iron, curling irons it's an awesome heat protector which help prevents damaged dry hair. Lastly, this is oil is great for adding other EOs for hair growth.
As it pertains to skin it protects elasticity and collagen and aids to tighten and tone the skin, high in Vitamin E, EFAs, and Omega 6. Regulates the production sebum and naturally stimulates skin tissue rejuvenation.

Ginger Root Oil

May be applied to the scalp and hair on its own or combined with another oil (argan, olive, coconut, jojoba.) Ginger increases circulation, combats dandruff, stimulates hair follicles to promote growth of new and existing hair. A good recipe for preparing ginger root can be found here.

Jojoba Oil

Jojoba Oil can be used with all hair and /or skin types. Most beneficial for extremely damaged or breaking hair, this carrier oil is considered a wax and not an oil. For hair that is over processed and damaged due to flat irons curling irons and other heat apparatus. The healing qualities of this carrier oil most promising. Jojoba oil can be applied directly to the hair, skin or scalp for restorative means. By adding EO for the type of hair and issue your client has this combination will begin the healing process. Jojoba oil can be used with any hair and skin type. Extremely damaged or breaking hair will benefit from the healing qualities of jojoba oil. This truly is one of the best base oils for hair loss due to breakage. The oil can be applied as described before apply in small amounts to the skin. Applying to the face will help prevent hair dye stains when dye is applied. This is a wax. See chart in chapter twelve.

Lanolin (Wax)
Has deep moisturizing effects, this locks in moisture, this is an emollient. Very greasy and thick, this is a byproduct of wool it's from a lamb and is classified as a wax not an oil or liquid. It melts at 100° F. this is best for dry hair products and dry skin.

Olive Oil or Extra Virgin Olive Oil
The Carrier oil is a great asset for faster hair growth. The essential ingredients of olive oil, is Vitamin D, E, & B (niacin and biotin). This oil is known to get rid of bald patterns of the scalp. Using olive oil infused with other EO that stimulates hair growth a notice of regrowth is possible. Plus, with daily use and by massaging this oil into the scalp hair growth is inevitable. Many hair experts regard olive oil as the best oil for hair loss can be used as a deep moisturizing treatment and to promote hair growth. Vitamin E in olive oil helps to improve blood flow to the scalp, which in turn stimulates hair growth. When it comes to its usage, a carrier oil such as jojoba oil is added to olive oil and then it is applied on the scalp. Look for Cold-pressed Olive Oil.

Please Note: This oil is great for Caucasian hair; it is a dry oil.

Pomegranate Seed Oil
One of the best herbs for thinning hair is this herb. This known to everyone as the "miracle" herb. With the punicic acid being the main ingredient that revitalizes the hair it also makes it shiny and thick. It proves as a protector against harsh products and other damaging environmental chemicals. This oil is very thick and can be mixed with other Carrier oils.

Peanut Oil
What binds this oil to hair is the chain of EFA. These EFAs are known as Omega 3•6•9 (oleic acid (omega 9 fatty acid), linoleic acid (omega 6 fatty acid), omega 3 fatty acids). Both oleic and linoleic acid, are important for

life threatening cell functions and the deficiency of either of these can lead to brittle or dry hair. We need both Omega 9 and 6 to fully function for Omega 3 to work. These three together allows the hair to grow and be healthy and allow for the scalp to stay moisturized and hydrated.
Being full of beneficial vitamins and nutrients Vitamin A has retinol in it. This has proven to be a cell rejuvenator and a cell recovery. This vitamin is also an excellent antioxidant but if you are deficient in this vitamin this can lead to dry hair and scalp even brittle hair. Adding this oil to the hair is an excellent moisturizer, it is naturally fortified with Vitamin E therefore it nourishes hair and will reverse damaged hair. Being full of other vitamins including Vitamin D which in turn prevents premature gray and dry scalp and promotes beautiful shiny healthy hair. This oil causes healthy hair because of it is richness in vitamins. This is oil is the best for hair & skin care products. Note: if you are allergic to peanuts stay away from this oil. For hair loss, it's been known for Vitamin D to prescribed to stop even reverse hair loss.

Safflower Oil
Safflower oil protects hair, nourishes hair follicles, moisturizes, and stimulates blood circulation to promote hair growth and thickness. And it is extremely beneficial for natural hair and for dry damage chemically treated hair.

Sesame Oil
This oil is known to be one of the best oils for hair treatments. Being extracted from seed this oil is extremely lubricating and nourishing. It is great for the scalp and for growing healthy hair. It naturally has Vitamin E and B complex plus necessary minerals, magnesium calcium phosphorus and protein that will strengthen the hair from the roots to the ends... to make the hair appear darker this oil is great. It is known to prevent and treat premature gray hair.

This oil not only promotes healthy hair growth, but it promotes it by increasing the scalp circulation and penetrates deeps within the scalp and hair strand shafts. When you have chemical damage or over processed hair this is the best oil to use in penetrates deep within each individual hair shaft that causes the hair to be restored.

When anti-bacterial measures are needed like to treat head lice or to deal with fungal infections like dandruff this oil mixed with the appropriate EO will cure the problem. Lastly this oil acts as an UV RAY blocker. Using the oil on the scalp prevents further damage from the sun.

Shea Butter
This butter is found in Africa from a tree called the Kotschy tree Karite`nuts. This is a heavy oil/butter but its benefits are amazing. This butter comes a nut that offer tremendous amounts of moisture to the hair and skin. This butter helps reduce dandruff, soothes the scalp and maintains a great shine on the hair.

Shea butter is a natural conditioner for hair, but this is also known to heal burns and injuries, and dispose of stretch marks and surgical marks, dermatitis. Apart from medicinal uses, some of the most common uses for Shea butter include using this as a natural moisturizer for your body and face, and as a conditioner for dry hair. It performs like a sealant and protectant against harmful UV rays, the environment, heat and styling tools.

Sunflower
This oil is a natural conditioner and moisturizer, it is full of minerals, vitamins and fatty acids it truly promotes healthy growing hair. This oil gives lots of shine because it penetrates deep into the cuticles of the hair shaft. Peanut oil is excellent in preventing hair loss, baldness and different types of alopecia. This oil can be used directly on the scalp or combined with other carrier oils and beneficial EOs.

This oil lessens the fizziness, reduces dryness and makes the hair easy to deal with manage.

CHAPTER 12

Essential Oils

The EOs can be applied on dry or toweled dry hair, and even applying it to hair in warm weather (to avoid the sun damaging rays) is an option. The most common way to make use of EOs hair care is to gently heat up your chosen EO (not too hot!) and apply it to your hair, gently massaging it into the scalp. Petroleum based oils nullifies EO properties

Lavender oil is an anti-inflammatory, anti-bacterial, anti-fungal, and antiseptic making it one of the most useful topical treatments for treating hair loss and other scalp ailments. Lavender oil increases circulation, promotes new hair growth, and helps to balance natural oil production of the scalp.

Note: Add lavender oil to olive or jojoba oil.

Peppermint oil is moisturizing, anti-fungal, and anti-inflammatory. When applied to the scalp, peppermint oil moisturizes skin and soothes irritation caused by chemical, microbial, and environmental damage. Peppermint also increases blood flow and stimulates follicles to grow new hair at an accelerated rate.

Note: Try this formula for a refreshing peppermint and jojoba scalp treatment.

Rosemary Essential Oil is one of the premier hair growth enhancing EOs. Rosemary is found in many hair and scalp. Its rumored to increase cellular metabolism, thereby stimulating healthy hair growth. Use the Verbenone type if regenerative properties are desired (may be most useful for supporting treatment of hair loss). Successfully used in alopecia aerate treatment. Rosemary oil is great for stimulating hair follicles for hair growth, preventing hair loss and graying, preventing dandruff, strengthening hair, and boosting shine.

Thinning hair tends to hold in more dirt and toxins; rosemary EO is great for cleansing and it also contains loads of vitamin B, iron and calcium. It has been used for thousands of years as a remedy for thinning and brittle hair, plus it has been scientifically proven to prevent premature graying.

Rosemary EO should be diluted with a carrier oil (such as extra virgin olive oil) before use. Use in formula at.5 - 2%.

ESENTIAL OILS & HERBS
Listed Below Are Common Herbs and Oils Used for Hair Care

ESSNTIAL OIL	PRIMARY PROPERTIES	HAIR TYPE & BENEFITS
ARNICA	Anti-inflammatory, antibacterial soothing & stimulant.	Oily hair. Promotes growth, stimulate follicles, stronger roots, natural sheen, split ends, increase circulation, premature gray
BASIL	Stimulant, Fragrance.	Oily hair. Promotes growth, stimulates circulation, high sheen
BLACK PEPPER	Stimulant	
BENZOIN	Antiseptic, deodorant, anti-inflammatory, disinfectant.	Great for oily hair, soothes open wounds, great aroma therapy ingredient.
BERGAMOT	Citrus, circulation, stimulant, disinfectant, antibiotic, sedative (soothes nerves), assists in fading scars and marks	Oily Hair type.
CEDARWOOD OIL	Antiseptic, astringent, antifungal.	Fine to normal hair types. Stimulates the scalp and follicles ; treats dandruff, promotes hair growth, normalize dry and oily hair and scalp.
		Fine to normal haïr types, offres

ESSNTIAL OIL	PRIMARY PROPERTIES	HAIR TYPE & BENEFITS
CHAMOMILE	Sedative, sheen.	golden highlights, soothes inflamed scalp, helps alleviate psoriasis, offers sheen.
CLARY SAGE	Antifungal, stimulant, circulation.	All hair types, Dandruff treatment, itchy scalp, promotes hair growth, stimulates scalp.
EUCALYPTUS	Anitmicrobial, antifungal, soothing, stimulant, fragrance.	Problematic hair types. Dandruff, itchy scalp.
GERANIUM	Fragrant, medicinal, astringent.	Oily hair types. Strengthen hair.
GRAPEFRUIT	Citrus, antiseptic, antifungal.	Oily hair.
LAVENDAR	Antimicrobial, antifungal, soothing, stimulant, fragrance.	All hair types. Itchy, dandruff, balance natural hair/scalp oils, deep conditions hair, soothes scalp, promotes growth, shiny hair.
LEMON	Citrus, stimulant, antifungal, disinfectant.	Oily hair types, offers golden highlights, treatment for dry scalp, dandruff, balance natural scalp oils.
LEMONGRASS	Citrus, stimulant, antifungal, disinfectant., antibacterial.	Oily hair types, slows scalp oil production.
MYRRH	Anti-inflammatory, sedative, antifungal.	Dry hair types, Hair treatment for dry scalp, dandruff.
PATCHOULI	Anti-inflammatory, sedative, antifungal, antiseptic.	Oily hair, dandruff treatment.
PEPPERMINT	Stimulant, astringent.	Dry hair, promotes growth by stimulating circulation.
ROASEMARY	Antiseptic, stimulant, antifungal, astringent.	Oily hair, dandruff treatment, promotes hair growth, stimulates roots.
SAGE	Antifungal, antimicrobial, antibacterial.	Problematic hair, clarifies scalp, beneficial for for psoriasis.
SANDALWOOD	Anti-inflammatory,	Dry hair, skin and fragrance.

ESSNTIAL OIL	PRIMARY PROPERTIES	HAIR TYPE & BENEFITS
	sedative, skin healing, antibacterial.	
SEA BUCKHORN	Antioxidant, regenerative.	
TEA TREE	Antifungal, emollient, disinfectant, antibacterial, antiviral, antimicrobial, expectorant.	Oily hair, treatment for dry scalp, dandruff, and lice.
THYME	Antiseptic, stimulant, tonic.	Stimulates blood flow, invigorates scalp, stimulates hair growth.
YANG YLANG	Antiseptic, stimulant.	Oily hair, dandruff treatment, soothing, stimulates hair growth.

Note: **These statements have not been evaluated by the Food and Drug Administration. Products and information on EOs are not intended to diagnose, treat, cure or prevent ANY disease. A decision to use/not use this information is the sole responsibility of the reader. Please see your doctor or health care professional for medical evaluation for yourself or your animals.**

There are other oils that benefit the use of EO:

Absolutes — The purest form of EOs obtained from plants (usually flowers) and that are used in formulas to make natural hair and skin products use these ingredients as a natural fragrance additive. These oils are usually thick, but very useful.

Agar Agar – This comes from the sea; known sea vegetables are mostly beneficial for natural products to blend oil and water together. This is a natural thickener when used properly. It offers antioxidants as well.

Aloe Vera — This is a plant from the succulent family. The plant offers high moisturizing properties and is known for many uses in hair care products. It can be purchased in powder, gel, or liquid form. It is known to smooth the skin and keep it soft, it is an anti-inflammatory, and is an excellent treatment for sunburns.

CHAPTER 13

Essential Oil (EO) Properties

Definition of EO Properties

- Antidepressant - Uplifting to the mind and spirit, alleviates depression (basil, bergamot, chamomile, geranium, jasmine, lavender, patchouli, rose, ylang ylang)

- Anti-fungal - Helps destroy fungus (lavender, myrrh, rosemary, tea tree)

- Anti-inflammatory- Reduces inflammation (basil, chamomile, frankincense)

- Anti-microbial/Antiseptic - Helps prevent the growth of bacteria. All EOs are antiseptic to a certain degree, with probably the most effective being (bergamot, eucalyptus, juniper)

- Antiviral - Counteracts the effects of viruses (cinnamon, eucalyptus, lavender, tea tree)

- Astringent - Causes skin tissue to contract, so good for toning skin (frankincense, geranium, peppermint, rosemary)

- Bactericidal - Helps destroy bacteria (clary sage, lemon, tea tree)
- Cephalic - Stimulating for the head and mind (basil, peppermint, rosemary)

- Deodorant - Works against and masks body odor (benzoin, bergamot, eucalyptus, lavender, patchouli)

- Detoxicant - Helps eliminate or reduce toxic substances (black pepper, juniper)

- Diuretic - Helps increase the production of urine (black pepper, chamomile, eucalyptus, geranium, juniper, lavender, rosemary)

- Rubefacient - Stimulates circulation locally and so causes redness of the skin (black pepper, eucalyptus, juniper, rosemary)

- Sedative - Has a soothing and calming effect (Bergamot, chamomile, frankincense, geranium, jasmine, juniper, lavender, patchouli, rose, ylang ylang)

- Stimulant - Has a invigorating action on the body and circulation (black pepper, eucalyptus, peppermint, rosemary, tea tree)

- Tonic - Tones the body generally, or in one area. Can be mildly stimulating and has a restorative effect (black pepper, chamomile, frankincense, geranium, jasmine, juniper, lavender, patchouli, peppermint, rose)

- Vulnerary - When applied externally heals cuts, sores and open wounds (benzoin, bergamot, chamomile, eucalyptus, frankincense, geranium, juniper, lavender, rosemary, tea tree)

CHAPTER 14

Hair Treatments

EOs can be thought of as the 'active ingredients' in your formulas.

Choose one or more and add them at the recommended concentrations to the carrier oil(s). Use the essential oils in chapter 12 for a guideline to match which EO blends well with one another. You'll often find adding EO of Lavender, Chamomile, Rosemary and Tea Tree in shampoos and conditioners makes a nice herbal shampoo. These particular EOs positively support the health of the scalp and hair follicles. Remember to choose the best EO and carrier oil(s) for your scalp issue, based on your hair type, see Chapter 2. Make or Mix the formulas in small batches and use immediately and keep in the refrigerator. Remember to follow simple directions this will help you create a most effective formula for your client.

Things to consider when blending EOs for Hair & Scalp Treatments

- Choose the appropriate essential and carrier oils for the clients scalp treatment.
- Make sure you like the aroma of the individual oils as well as the blend of oils.
- Make sure you like the fragrance of the oils!
- Try to choose oils that have synergy. (Synergy: Refer to Chapters 11, 12 and 13)

Record keeping is of the upmost important. Keep a record of every drop and mix while blending hair and scalp treatments. It is totally upsetting to make the perfect formula and can't remember the cups, ounces, millilters used to make this awesome product.

When blending EOs, it is a good idea to **keep a record** of mixes that you like. It is very frustrating when you have found a wonderful aroma.........but just can't quite remember which oils you used and in what quantities! This has happened to me so many times. I mixed the PERFECT formula but didn't write it down…

Likewise, if a blend turns out to be pungent, or irritating to the skin you will want to make sure you don't make the same mistake again!!!!

EOs can be classified under heading like floral, citrus, spicy, woody, green, resins. The oils in the same heading blend well together but this still is based on your nose and what you like.

When EOs are blended together they produce a healing effect. When combined it's a stronger effect and will offer better results because of its concentration. This is known as good synergy in the Aromatic world. Blending oils with the same properties offer very good benefits.

Please Note: This is only a suggested guide and tips for blending EOs together.

When creating a formula in the U.S. if the ingredient makes up 1% of the product ingredients does not have to be listed. Just the key components.

But let's keep it simple- think of putting the ingredients into three categories.

Find the EOs you need for an issue you may have. List in order the issue then find the EOs that are known to address that issue. Next find the carrier oil that complements the EOs and that is beneficial to the issue. List how much of the product you are interested in making. Start with the size of the container and start there.

Example:

- Start with a 2 oz., bottle
- Choose the EOs for the issue at hand

- Choose the carrier oil. See charts on pages 146-148.
- Add the EOs remember to count how many drops you used
- Perform a test trial to see how the formula works on your skin Log and document the results. You many increase the formula.

- ✓ ***Functional Ingredients-*** These ingredients have the effect, feel or the appearance on your hair or skin. Whatever product you make it needs to have at least one Functioning ingredient in it.
- ✓ ***Aesthetic Ingredients-*** These are the most prevalent and necessary ingredients. These ingredients make the product a product, these are the solvents, thickeners, preservatives, pH adjusters. These ingredients are for the benefit of your hair/skin, it's for the benefit of ingredients.
- ✓ ***Claims Ingredients-*** These ingredients are why you will use this product. These ingredients that create a story about the product. They imply what this product will do, what it does. These ingredients normally are listed last in the list of ingredients.

Make a precise list of how much you used per ingredient for every formula.

- ✓ What EOs are you using. list them
- ✓ What carrier oil did you put with the EO list it.

What other ingredient was used for example preservatives fragrance?

Dilutions for Scalp & Hair Treatments using EO'S:

.5% *is* ***four drops of EO*** *to* ***one ounce of Carrier Oil***

1**% Essential Oil** or ***8 drops of EO*** per one ***ounce*** of ***Carrier Oil***

These are estimated percentages **TABLE 2**

Percent %	E O Drops	ml.	Ounces
.25%	2	2.5	0.084535
.5%	4	5	0.169070
1%	8	10	0.338140
Percent %	E O Drops	ml.	Ounces
2%	16	20	0.676280
3%	24	30	1.014420
4%	32	40	1.352560
5%	40	50	1.690701
10%	80	100	3.381402
Ounces	Gram	Ounces	Gram
1	28.34952	48	1360.777
2	56.6990	64	1814.369
3	85.04856	128	3628.738
4	114.3980		
8	226.7961		
10	283.4952		
12	340.1942		
16	459.5923		
24	680.3885		
36	1020.5828		

To define treatment in my words is to treat a condition that is leading to a major issue, it is to prevent any further damage or outbreak to an occurring issue that is causing an issue, irritation or problem.

The British define it as:

n.

1. The application of medicines, surgery, psychotherapy, etc, to a patient or to a disease or symptom

Treatment in Medicine Expand

treatment treat·ment (tr ē t'm ə nt)
n.
Administration or application of remedies to a patient or for a disease or an injury; medicinal or surgical management; therapy. (The Amerian Heritage Science Dictionary, 2016)

Based on these definitions mine is close: We define our world to suit us as needed without hurt harm or creating disaster to anyone.

Listed in the next pages are proven treatments for the benefit of helping you. These treatments have been tested on numerous clients over the years with phenomenal results. We are not making any claims nor have any of the treatments been tested or approved by the FDA (who wants to go through 8-10 years of scrutiny and unnecessary headache when what God made/created has already been proven and declared GOOD!!)

Take the time to completely read all ingredients become familiar with sizes, herbal names and definitions. When mixing products, treatments or formulas know that there is nothing new under the sun, but what you create claim it.

Test all formulas on yourself if possible before using them on others, strangers, family members. When using treatments that you formulate make sure you are aware of their allergies.

Get to know as much as you can about your issue begin with your dietary habits, lifestyle issues, deep personal issues that may be affecting or causing the hair loss if this is your issue…

In making products and formulas there are basic equipment that is needed and necessary when making natural products/formulas. This is to name a few necessary items to be successful.

EQUIPMENT NEEDED:

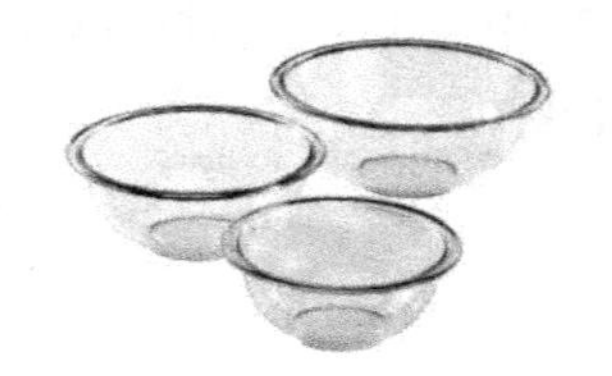

GLASS PYREX BOWLS

RUBBER SPATULA

MEASURING SPOONS

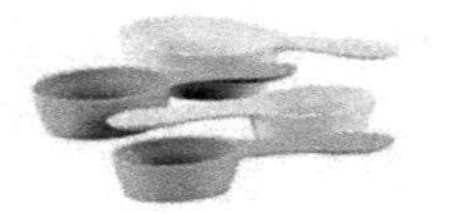

MEASURING SPOONS

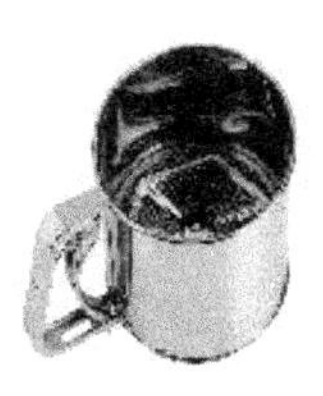

SIFTERS

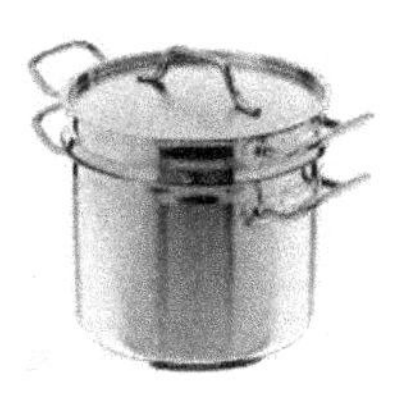

DOUBLE BOILER POT SET

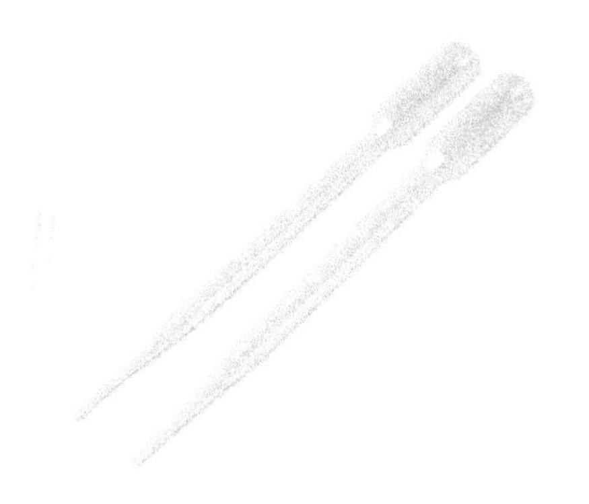

PIPETTES

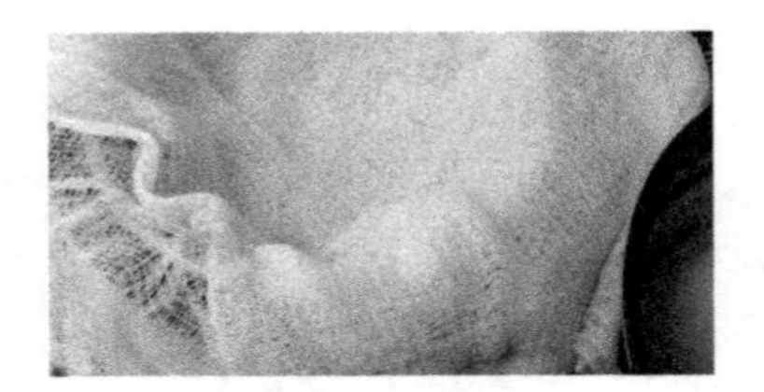

NATURAL CHEESE CLOTHS

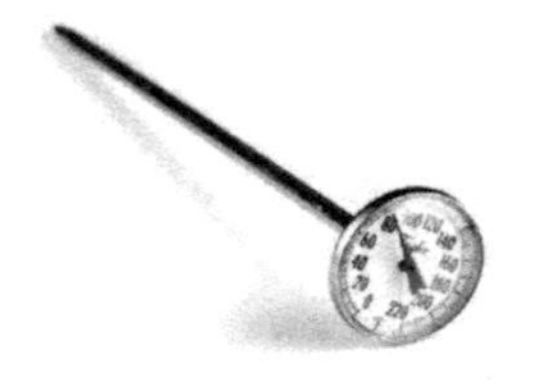

FOOD THERMOMETER

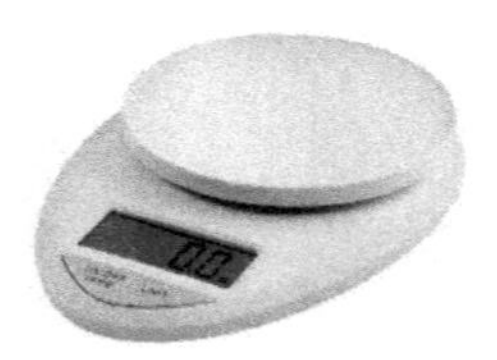

FOOD SCALE

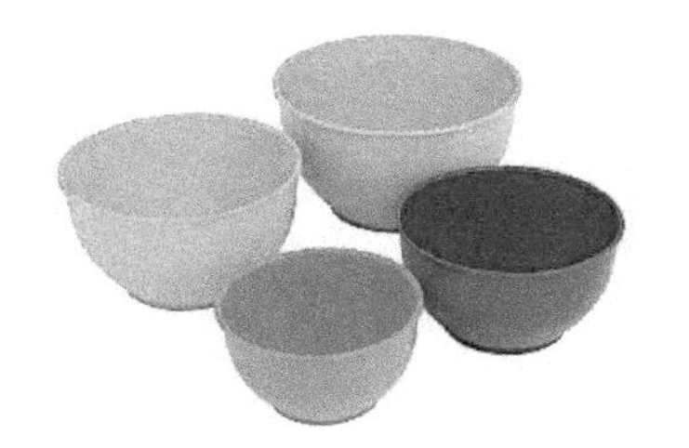

MIXING BOWLS

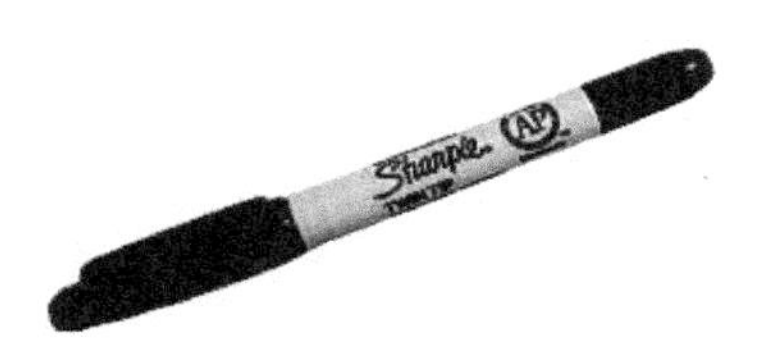

MARKERS

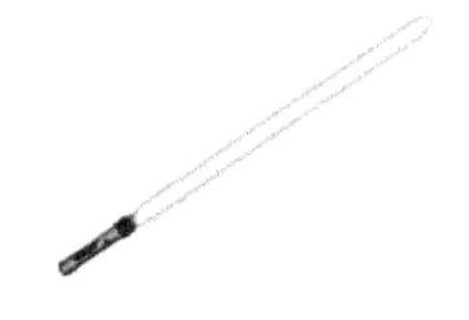

GLASS ROD (SPATULA)

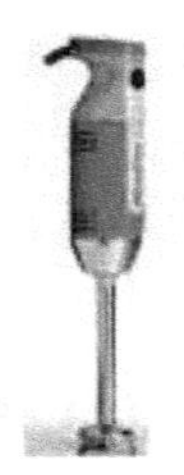

HAND MIXER

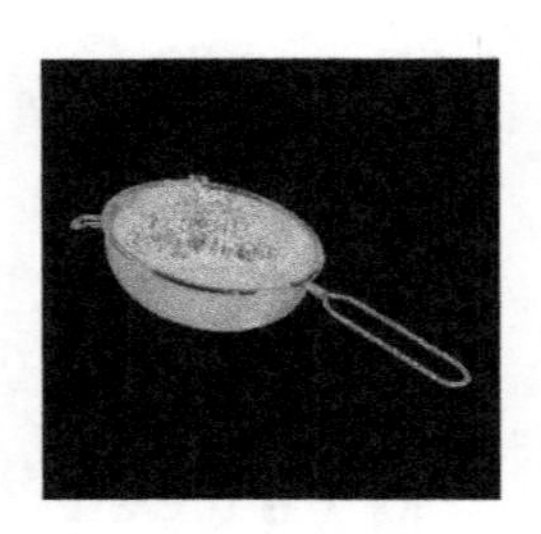

STRAINER

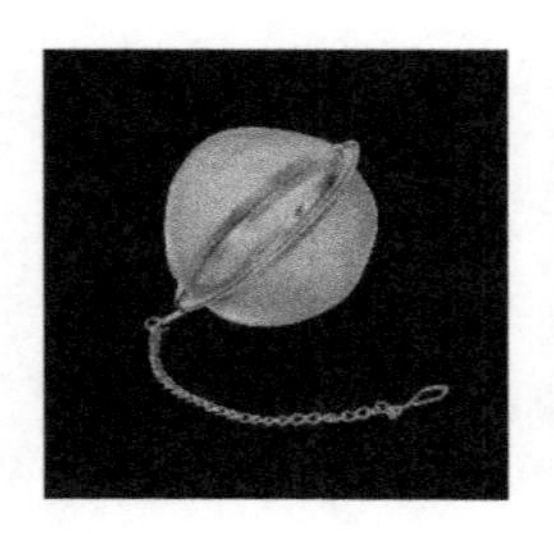

MESH TEA BALL

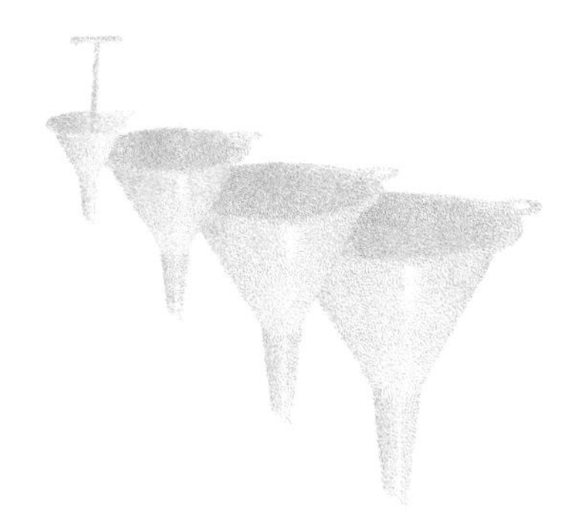

FUNNELS

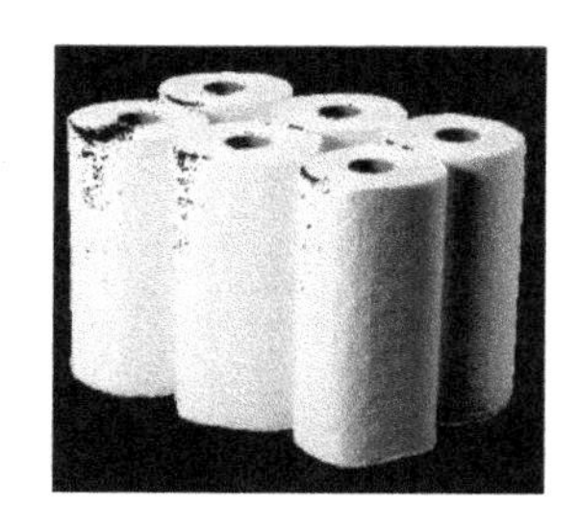

PAPER TOWELS

Hair & Scalp Treatments

Oils for Hair Growth Use Alone or Combined

Carrot Root Oil (**To stimulate hair follicles)**

Mix with:

1) 1 oz. or (57 gr) Jojoba Oil
    a. 1 oz Basix™
    b. Carrot Root Oil
    c. Use at 1 - 3% (1.70 gr)

2) 4 oz Amber Bottle or dark colored bottle
    a. 2oz (57 gr) Safflower Flower Oil
    b. 1 oz Basix™
    c. Use Carrot Seed Oil at.5 - 2%(up to 1.70 gr)

3) Use with 4oz Bottle
    a. 1 oz Grapeseed
    b. 1 oz Jojoba OI
    c. .5 oz Basix™
    d. Use at.5 - 1% Combination of Carrot Seed Oil
    e. Lavender 4 d. (make sure you use a total of 10 dr per this formula based on how many ounces it is using)
    f. Rosemary
    g. Thyme 2 dr. (you can mix or change, dr=drops)

4) Use a 4oz. jar or bottle (coconut oil cools it becomes a solid)
    a. Coconut Oil (Fractionated)
    b. 2 oz (gr) Coconut Oil
    c. 1oz Basix™
    d. 1.5 oz (45.5 gr) Chamomile Oil or herb (fresh herbs)

5) Clary Sage
    a. Use with 4 oz bottle
    b. 1 oz Sesame Oil
    c. 1oz Basix™
    1.5 oz Clary Sage

6) Clove Fresh or Oil
    a. Use with 4oz Bottle
    b. 3 oz Safflower Oil
    c. .5 Clove
    d. .5 Black Pepper

7) Tea Tree Oil
    a. 2oz Dark Amber Bottle
    b. 3% of Tea Tree EO Use 1-6 drops in 2 oz oil.
    c. By adding 3% EO to a carrier oil base. Massage into the scalp and wrap in warm towels for two.

To prevent gray hair

4oz Dark Amber Bottle
1.5 oz Carrier Oil for your type hair
1 oz Use another carrier oil for your hair type (dandruff prone, thinning)
5 dr. Rosemary EO.
5 dr. Sage E. O.
1 5 dr. Burdock Root
5 dr. Licorice

Warm Carrier oil to normal temperature (120°). Add let cool add EOs. Seal bottle and let sit for 24-48 hours then apply as often as needed

.

Protein & Hair Treatments

"**Protein doesn't moisturize hair**," says Jose Eber Salon senior stylist Paul Anthony. It strengthens it. Women tend to use it more than they should, which causes their hair to break, become weak and even brittle". This leads us to the common misconception about protein treatments - oftentimes, we do assume it *will* hydrate our hair when it's dried out, when this is just the opposite, what we should be using are products with humectant (moisturizing) ingredients like shea butter, sesame oil, oils and jojoba.[15]

There are several different types of protein ingredients found in hair care products.

To list a few

- ✓ wheat proteins,
- ✓ keratin,
- ✓ soy protein,
- ✓ silk amino acids.

The hair is made up of a tough fibrous keratin protein. Protein assist to strengthen the tresses and allow the hair to grow strong and long. Note: if too much protein is used or to many treatments are performed the hair will turn dry and brittle and healthy hair is out the window.

There's an easy way to figure out what your hair needs- if it seems to lack luster, on the dry side.

- ❖ **After you wash your hair (and it's still wet), grab a strand of it and pull a one-inch section apart between your fingers.**
- ❖ **If the hair breaks apart right away, it needs more moisture.**
- ❖ **If it stretches out far, with or without breaking, then it needs more protein.**
- ❖ **Hair that has a perfect balance of moisture and protein will stretch just a little and then return to its normal length without breaking.**

---

[15] http://www.newbeauty.com/

If you determine that your hair is in need of a protein treatment, choose a product that is beneficial for your hair type and condition. Follow the product directions. Then follow the 3 C's process. Do this until there is improvement (once a week is fine.) Oils won't hurt the hair.

When the following chemical services are performed on a regular basis having routine protein treatments is a plus in having healthy hair. Chemical services could be any of the following: color, relaxer, perms, texturize (this product is still a relaxer just milder), keratin treatments and heat style (roller set, flat iron, hot comb, blow dryer).

Keratin Myths

Keratin are from amino acids combined with the other properties of amino acids. Depending upon the combination and differences and intensities of the of amino acids defines if it's a hair, skin, hoof (yes animal feet), nails, teeth, this fiber can be hard or flexible. Keratin is a very strong fibrous protein. What is so unimaginative it that this amino acid is dead fibers. Daily the body sheds old cell which brings forth new cell and the old cells push the new cells out. With this type of Keratin, that is hair type of Karatin, we strive to keep the hair well moisturized and conditioned. In doing this the hair will remain stronger longer and healthy, waiting for the new keratin to arrive as (hair growth). Our hair strands, finger nails and teeth (this is why dentist tell us once the enamel is destroyed its gone), this is why keratin type cells sheds so much. Our skin, sheds our finger nails, our hair sheds but at the same time is being renewed with new ones.

When protein treatments are properly administered, this will not hurt/damage the hair. Even for clients who wear their hair chemical free or "all natural", it is important to moisturize the hair when performing protein treatments. There must be a balance so your hair will not dry out or become brittle. Thus, reversing the healthy hair care regimen.

For all natural hair protein treatments comes in various strengths. This type of hair may choose a milder protein treatment without worrying about other serious issues that may stem from intense stronger protein treatment that is used for other seriously damaged hair.

* Basic may be purchased on our website: **www.RXestoratives.com**

With the use of chemicals: relaxer, perm, color, straighteners (Keratin) contributes to the weakness of hair strands, these types of processes and services damages the outer cuticle layer of the hair.

Protein treatments work to restore the hair shaft back up. A lot of day to day hair care techniques does create damage to the hair cuticle or outer layer of the hair shaft. If your client has any of these signs of dry, damaged brittle hard hair, find the protein treatment regimen for your client hair type and problems soon as possible.

- **Elasticity Test**

  Healthy hair in good condition can stretch without breaking, normally. Hair in good condition can stretch under normal conditions without breaking. To perform an elasticity test, follow the steps below.

- Comb thru the hair find long strands of hair to perform the test:
- Pull the strand of hair, see if it easily snaps back without breaking.
- If it does, your hair is in good shape.
- If you stretch the hair strand it and it breaks easily, a Protein treatment is needed in your hair.

Formulas for elasticity test treatments:

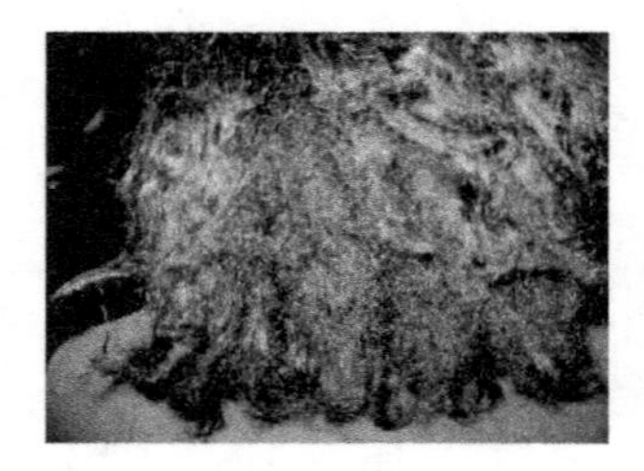

Over processed hair is considered damage hair. When hair is over processed due to chemicals, it can feel and look like straw when it's wet. When the hair is dry, it may feel like a rough like straw or hay. Although ethnic hair is not the normal soft silky type of hair texture a straw like feel is not the norm.

When the hair is severely damaged, all the moisture is completely gone. It's not the average hair shedding, this the norm…normally we lose 100-200 strands per day but this like when your clients experiences hair breakage and severe shedding. A protein treatment is necessary as soon as possible. This is a true sign that the hair is very weak and brittle.

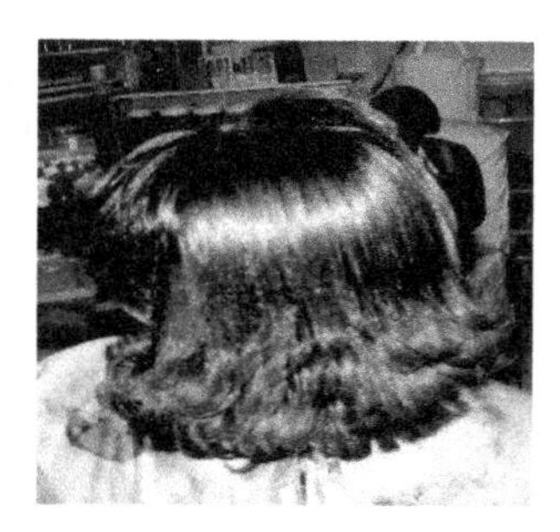

For severe damage hair, a protein treatment at this point may or may not help. Be assured that a cut may be necessary at this time but be reassured that the hair will grow back with the proper care and the proper hair & scalp treatments it will grow back healthy and strong especially with a Holistic Herbal approach to hair care. There are proven treatments that can begin the treatment process for damaged over processed hair.

TREATMENT

- Apply 1-2 oz of product all oil all over hair, massage in well, place plastic cap for 20 minutes with or without heat. This depends on damage
- Rinse hair
- RX Baking Soda Treatment Make a paste with water follow with a
- Conditioner
- Shampoo
- Condition
- ACV30 Leave-In Conditioner
- Style as usual
- For your next treatment, Follow the above steps but AVOID THE BAKING SODA TREATMENT!!!!

Retail Product for purchase is: RX® Oils of Nature*, RX® ACV30*, RX® Glossifier* these products are good if you have Chemicals in your hair. For Natural Clients: RX® Tress Pomade*, RX® Oils of Nature*, RX® HotCombNBottle*.

Treatment: Protein

One Treatment		Second Treatment	
Coconut Milk	½ c	Avocado Butter	2 oz
Coconut Oil	2 Tbsp	RX® Oils of Nature	1 oz
RX® Oils of Nature	1 Tbsp		
Warm Honey	2 Tbsp		

Types of Conditioner Formulas For Dry and Damaged Hair:

INGREDIENTS:

- 2 ounces' aloe vera gel
- 1/2 teaspoon olive/avocado/jojoba oil
- 2 ounces' organic apple cider vinegar
- 1 ounce powdered milk

Combine ingredients in a bowl and apply to clean, wet hair. Allow formula to remain on hair for 10 to 15 minutes, then rinse well with warm water.

Marshmallow Root

1 cup Marshmallow Root

Boil dried marshmallow for about fifteen minutes then strain to extract mucilage which can then be combined with your favorite home conditioner.

Protein Conditioners

Protein conditioners do not change the hair structure, but as with protein rinses they add some body as well as imparting shine and enabling easier brushing and combing. Unfortunately, protein conditioners are often advertised as somehow repairing damaged hair and keratins. ***This is not true to any significant degree***. Hair above the skin is dead, it is chemically inert and insoluble. It is extremely difficult to get the keratins in hair fiber to chemically react with anything and certainly your average protein conditioner is not able to.

Protein conditioners coat the hair fibers in a layer of proteins that make the hair ***look thicker***, it's a perception thing. Protein conditioners are useful for adding body and allow thin/fine hair to appear thicker. If the outer cuticle is damaged the protein conditioner assist in filling in the gaps. By performing this treatment, the hair will be smoother, less tangle and should have a natural shine to it. *However, this does not actually improve hair strength, protein conditioners just plaster over the surface, and they do not significantly penetrate the hair and improve the internal* *fiber structure. The effects of protein conditioners are a temporary fix. Regular care and treatments are still a must.*

NOTE: Some popular protein conditioners contain keratins and most advertisers make suggestions if you notice they NEVER MAKE DIRECT CLAIMS about what a product will do they only hint or make insinuations.

Preserves Hair Protein

For hair that needs a natural protein plant based conditioner try Deep conditioning the hair once every 2 weeks. This is very good for Type 2C hair.

- 1 oz. Raw Shea Butter
- Medium Avocado
- 1 Lg Egg (for protein)
- 2 tsp. Bentonite Clay

Directions:
In a bowl, soften Shea Butter <u>Do Not Heat</u>, get the Shea Butter to room temperature (like if you would leave it outside in the sun for a few minutes). Cut the Avocado in half remove the seed and the skin, beat the egg then add all the ingredients together until it has a nice consistency. It may be a little lumpy that's fine just mix all ingredients well. Add the clay once all the other ingredients are blended completely.
Apply to hair with cotton around the head add plastic cap. Allow your body heat to do the conditioning. Leave on for 45 minutes to an hour depending on the condition of the hair. When rinsing this treatment out ONLY use conditioner.

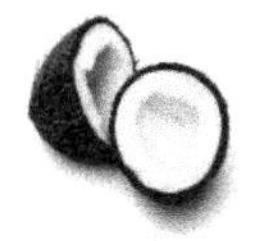

A major study was performed that compared Coconut Oils with Sunflower and mineral Oil, these are two most used oils in the cosmetic industry. The study concluded that out of the three oils coconut oil was the only oil that preserved protein in damaged or non-damaged hair.

The composition molecular size of Triglycerides found in coconut oil are able to penetrate the hair shaft which allows this oil to penetrate the hair and thus protects the hair from loss of protein. This oil allows the hair to be shiny and soft when used properly because it is absorbed deep within the shaft.

The sebaceous glad secrets oil which help to protect the scalp and hair making it waterproof like and not easily dry, damaged or brittle.

When using coconut as a hot oil treatment and for regular use (a product that has natural coconut oil in it) it the hair shaft is not only built up and stronger but the hair is healthier and shiny. When choosing to use, this oil follow the hair treatments directions. The longer it stays on the hair the healthier results you attain.

Consuming the oil is best by adding this oil as substitute for vegetable oil or canola oil or even olive oil this oil well produce great result all over for your hair skin and body.

FOR OILY HAIR

SHOCKING BUT NO CONDITIONER PERIOD!!!! You need to use volumizing products on hair that is oily and/or limp. If your hair is oily, then adding moisture back into your strands after shampooing isn't needed. However, if skipping conditioner altogether makes you uncomfortable, stay away from the products mentioned above: you may even try adding citrus EOs to your conditioner, for oily limp hair. Your key words when purchasing products is "volumizing," "light," "strengthening," or "balancing."

Using a shampoo that is clear is your best bet as well.

Use hydrating conditioner on slightly-to-moderately dry hair. If your hair isn't severely brittle or damaged, but feels a little on the dry side, switch to a product that advertises as

DAMAGED HAIR IN NEED OF REPAIR

For hair in need of repair find products that are labeled "damage repair" conditioner. If your hair is extremely dry and frizzy this product is best for you as well. For this kind of hair, you'll need to use more intensive oil based formulas.

Hair often becomes "damaged" and dried out by prolonged exposure to heat from daily styling tools like flat irons, curling irons, blow dryer ... but heat damage is not the only reason for extremely dry hair. At times hair become damage because of the upkeep or being un-kept.

Hair becomes unhealthy and dry, simply because your scalp has trouble producing enough oil to distribute throughout the strands. Either way, conditioners that advertise themselves as treatments for "damaged" hair will be effective on hair that's dry both because of heat exposure and natural causes.

The best approach for hair that is in need of repair, use the three C process:

- **Conditioner:** Use Conditioner as your FIRST SHAMPOO
- **Shampoo:** Use the proper Shampoo for your clients' hair
- **Conditioner:** Use the Conditioner again as your final wash
- Follow Up with a herbal **Leave-In Conditioner**.

1. Start with a **baking soda** treatment (found in the treatment section) Remember this is you first "cleanser"
2. Rinse the hair very good and when you are tied of rinsing rinse the hair more
3. Apply Conditioner that is specific for damaged hair
4. Do a quick cleanser (shampoo) Rinse thoroughly.
5. Condition again, Rinse the hair
6. Add Leave-in-Conditioner

Another added suggestion:

- Coconut oil is also an effective weekly treatment for extremely dry hair.

Find other oils that complement dry hair and perform a HOT OIL treatments for this type of hair.

Chemically treated hair regular conditioner reconstructors:

Ok for "relaxed" hair or leave-in conditioners (that are oil based) for relaxed hair. Many African American women love relaxed hair, it's easy to maintain and style. Though the process offer results that are unfavorable, with the right hair management the hair will grow and still be healthy. To avoid these issues DO NOT over shampoo the hair, use styling tools and excessive heat, lastly, do regular Hot Oil treatments and deep conditioning treatments* that are oil based. Shampoo for relaxed hair for added protection add a carrier oil to the shampoo and conditioner. Follow the RXHSW™ Three C process for conditioning and shampooing hair.

When using conditioning masks, remember to let the product soak into your hair for at least 10-15 minutes before rinsing it out, or else it won't have time to hydrate your hair effectively.

Do the hair mask made with Avocado and Honey

Start with a product build up remover

- ¼ c Apple Cider Vinegar
- 2 Tbsp. Honey
- 1 Lemon grated Lemon
- Warm Honey add to ACV, mix well.
- Grate the entire lemon peel to already mixed product.
- Apply product to the hair and wash the hair with both hands together rub hands in hair. Leave on hair for 15-20 minutes.
- Rinse the product out with cool water, do a quick conditioner rinse hair and style as usual. Follow up with a natural Leave-N-Conditioner. (ACV[30*])

- This mask removes product build up and will condition the hair plus leave the hair soft and shiny.

Then for conditioner do an Oil based Deep Conditioner treatment or a HOT OIL Treatment, use natural oils for this treatment, at least once per month. This is done to prevent breakage and brittle hair that leads to dryness.

Dry Dull Damaged Hair Treatment

If you feel like being daring, try this one:

Ingredients:

- 1 Whole Ripe Avocado
- 1 Tbsp Fresh Squeezed Lemon juice
- 1 tsp. Sea Salt
- 1 Tbsp. Castor Oil
- 1 Tbsp. Aloe Gel or Juice
- 2 Tbsp Warm Honey for oily Hair use Citrus Orange Honey

Cut Avocado in half place in bowl, glass or stainless steel. Mash Avocado add all the ingredients and blend until it's a smooth consistency, creamy like a thick lotion.

Apply all over to hair. Rub on hair for even distribution. Apply plastic cap, for an hour no heat is necessary your body heat is enough. Rinse product out of the hair with a quick conditioner. Add a Moisturizing Leave-In Conditioner. Style as usual.

Treat dandruff with light, fragrance-free conditioners. Dandruff is a scalp issue, not a hair issue; the skin on your scalp grows and dies at a faster rate than in people without dandruff, leaving an embarrassing flaky white residue in your hair and on your shoulders.[8] The shampoo you choose will have more of an effect on your dandruff than your conditioner, but there are still many products on the market geared toward treating this condition.

Look for lighter conditioners rather than high moisturizing or oil-heavy ones that can contribute to the problem on your scalp.[9]

Hair products with heavy fragrances often irritate the scalp, which leads to more itching, and more evidence of your dandruff on your clothes. Avoid heavily perfumed conditioners.

How to Condition Dry Hair

Conditioning is essential for great hair it allows the cuticles to close and makes the hair less frizzy more manageable to work with and shinier.

Doing it the RXHSW® way. Use a quarter sized (plus or minus, depending on how much hair you have) and rub product between both hands. Begin at the tips of your hair this prevents split ends. And work your way up to the scalp. Evenly apply conditioner over the entire head. Scrubbing at this point is necessary because this is acting like a "shampoo". At this point you might need to add a bit more product. Rinse the hair. Follow conditioner instructions for time to leave on the hair.
Note: the longer it says to stay on the hair the less alcohol it has in it.

Add shampoo, the shampoo for your type hair, we covered this in earlier chapters.

- ❖ Rinse the hair
- ❖ Then reapply Conditioner. At this point for normal hair if needed a plastic cap can be applied for 15 minutes, your body heat is enough heat needed. This allows the conditioner to absorb into the shaft.

- ❖ Finally rinse the conditioner out completely, scrub if you feel you need to.
- ❖ Follow with for oily type hair a citrus type Leave-in-Conditioner
- ❖ For Dry prone hair an Oil Base Leave-in-Conditioner
- ❖ For hair stimulating properties look for a Leave=in-Conditioner that has these ingredients in it or you can make it yourself. Give it a try.

Hair Tips:

- ✓ When brushing your hair out after shampoo, use a flat wide tooth comb to detangle your hair, not a normal round brush because it causes split ends, damages hair after shampoo the is wet and easy to break.
- ✓ Make sure to find a conditioner for your "**type hair** "and for oily prone scalp fine one that washes out completely because of the oils in conditioners, if all of the oil doesn't wash out, it'll end up on your face and back, which causes back acne and acne, which could possibly turn into scars.
- ✓ If more moisture is needed here is a little trick find a product used for curly hair, try because curly hair has more moisture type ingredients in it which allows them to manage their hair better.

Quick hair care tips

1) Try the natural way to Wash with hair that is dry, dull, damaged or even normal hair:

- ❖ Conditioner: Use Conditioner as your FIRST SHAMPOO
- ❖ Shampoo: Use the proper Shampoo for your clients' hair
- ❖ Conditioner: Use the Conditioner again as your final wash

- Follow Up with a herbal Leave-In Conditioner. Use the product that applies to the client current hair condition. Not all products are equal and is not suitable everyone. During the summer, you don't wear jackets and mittens and boots-you wear sandals and swim suits.

2) When shampooing, your hair cover every aspect of the scalp, my suggestion and only a suggestion to make sure you cover every corner of the scalp,

- start at the nape of neck
- work your way up above the ears then scrub the center
- [i] on the front of the scalp to finish up at the hair line
- then reverse don't scrub especially
- If the hair is naturally oily take time to rid the scalp of flakes. Rubbing the cuticle via washing the hair may cause the hair/scalp to flake more unless a treatment is performed.

3) If you have dry hair daily shampooing needs to be avoided. If you must, must shampoo your hair find a low pH sulfate free shampoo and conditioner (4-7pH). Hair fibers being frequently cleansed can be quite damaging. That why I strongly suggest the RXHSW® method 3C's (Condition, Cleanser, Conditioner). Excessive shampooing of the hair will strip away necessary oils that is needed on the shafts.

4) Read labels not only for food but for hair products as well. Look for strong oil stripping ingredients such as *sodium lauryl sulfate*. Sodium laureth sulfate is milder and some shampoos do away with sodium sulfate based detergents altogether.

MINERAL OIL & PETROLATUM, PEG, PROPYLENE GLYCOL, SODIUM LAURYL SUFATE (SLS) & SODIUM LAURETH SULFATE, (SOME OF THE NITROSATING AGENTS ARE: SLS, SLES, DEA, TEA, MEA). **DEA (diethanolamine) MEA (momoethnanolamine) TEA (triethanolamine): these are preservatives: IDAZOLIDINYL UREA and DMDM HYDANTOIN:**

5) If you have very dry hair, look for shampoos with humectants in them. African Americans have trouble with dull, difficult hair and may find a

variety of mild oil based products useful for application after washing. There is the potential for scalp irritation from the oils so pay close attention to how your clients scalp responds and avoid using them if you notice any side effects.

6) Use a separate conditioner. The all-in-one shampoo and conditioners is okay for average hair but they are not good for dry hair. Separate conditioner plus very mild shampoo is much superior to a combined product. Please note how to apply shampoo and Conditioner Apply conditioner in a milking fashion as with the shampoo. Perform the RXH&SW shampoo process.

7) If your you have dull, dry, problem hair using chemical processes (relaxers, perms, color) is definitely out. These types of salon chemical services contribute to the bonds in the hair being broken down. The hair has two layers the cuticle and cortex. These services will lead to permeant damage.

8) African American should avoid frequent chemicals services and especially when it pertains to relaxers hair straighteners and high lift hair color. African American hair has low sulfur protein content compared to high sulfur protein than found in Asian or Caucasian individuals.

9) Your genetic makeup plays a serious role in your hair. Having brittle hair must be treated with specific treatments found in the back of the manual. Sometimes even with our Western diet (foods we eat in America) incorporating supplements, vitamins can help to alter our hair. Remember what goes in is what comes out. There are vitamins and supplement that are hair specific. Supplements like Silica, Biotin, Folic Acid, magnesium - **Note**: you must take magnesium for the body to absorb certain supplement/vitamins. Also, more is not better do not over consume these supplements! Follow the manufacture daily use dosage.

10) Using the proper tools is always best. Use a boar's brush (natural bristle brush) for the hair for good results. Using a metal or wooden comb (hard to find though) plastic combs create too much static. Comb/Brush the hair from the root to the ends. Using these tips allows the hair to be very manageable.

11) In certain states like my state Florida it's hard to avoid sunlight. This is why we live here ☺...anyway if at all possible avoid constant direct sunlight, air pollution like working at a construction sites, train stations, high chemical based jobs. Having constant contact with these can breakdown the bonds of the roots of the hair (hair follicles) if you must be outdoors like mailmen/women cover the hair up...

Hot Oil Treatment

2 oz Castor Oil

1oz Sesame Oil

1oz Coconut Oil

Mix oils together warm in a double boiler. Heat up 120° F, Stir. Let cool then apply evenly all over hair. Place plastic cap over hair leave on for 30-45 minutes, Rinse with cool water, light conditioner, apply Oil based Leave-in Conditioner, for those with oily hair use citrus EO in Hot Oil Treatment.

Remedies for Dry Damaged Hair

Herbal Rinse May Help to Stop Hair Loss

Herbal rinses have been used for over hundreds of years. Herbal rinses will naturally soften hair, increase manageability, and restore shine and luster body and bounce. Herbal hair rinses provide you with a deep cleansing when the appropriate herbs are used for the rinse, they may lighten, darken or enhance your natural hair color. By using herbs that are known to soothe irritated hair and scalps (see the EO chart for more detail). They can prevent dandruff and may stimulate the scalp to increase growth.

Natural herbal rinses are nourishing and gentle for the scalp. They depend on herbs, EOs to promote a healthy scalp and stronger longer healthier hair. Plus, other ingredients especially synthetic ingredients can cause product build up and damage the hair.

Soap Nuts Liquid Recipe

- 15-20 soap nuts
- 1T Marshmallow Root
- 6 cups of water (plus more as you're boiling)
- Sterilized container to hold the liquid

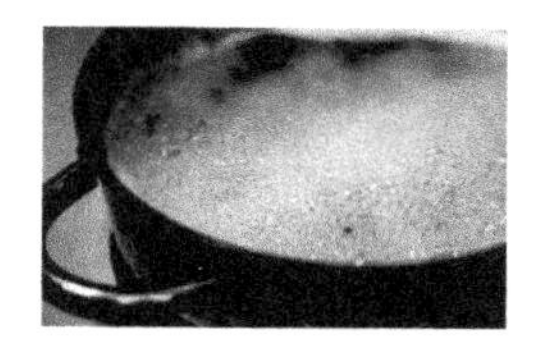

Boil the soap nuts in the four cups of water for about 20 minutes. Add another cup of water. Boil for ten minutes. Add another two cups of water and boil again for ten minutes. Add the marshmallow powder mix well. Strain the nuts from the liquid and store in the sterilized container. Now, as you're boiling the liquid, keep an eye on it. Otherwise, it will start to suds a little and might boil over. This happened the first time I made liquid. I took this picture right after the over boil. It's best to store the straight liquid in the refrigerator, or it will turn rancid after a while. Keep this in the refrigerator for 1-2 weeks.

Hot Oil & Transitioning Treatment

2 c. Apple Cider Vinegar

1 c. Distilled Water

30 dr. Rosemary E. O.*

30 dr. Sage E. O.*

These E. O. combined have been known to darken gray hair

*= Rxestoratives Hair & Skin Wellness Sell these items.

Do not immediately use Herbal Rinse. Let sit for 48-72 hours before use. Do not store for over 30 days.

Amla for Hair Growth

2 T. Amla powder

2 oz. Coconut Oil

2 oz. Castor Oil

Mix Amla powder with Castor oil and Coconut oil, warm oils to 80° F. Massage into the scalp. Leave on hair/ scalp overnight or use with heat for 20 minutes with plastic cap.

Damaged Soar Scalps

Thyme oil 20-30 drops and to the Carrier oil of your choice (sesame oil, sweet almond, etc.)

Warm oil not above 90 F. Let set for 48-72 hours before use

Place in dark glass bottle.

Place client in chair after **RXHSW®** shampoo method:

- Condition
- Shampoo
- Condition

This method ensures healthy hair from start to finish. If the hair is excessively dry, then start with a Hot Oil Treatment first. Find the appropriate Treatment for the clients' hair and scalp issue.

Head Lice

10 dr. Eucalyptus Oil

10 dr. Rosemary E O

5 dr. Tea Tree EO

3oz Sesame Oil

ground flax seeds boiled in water will form a soothing gel that can be applied to scalp and hair to moisturize skin, eliminate dandruff, stimulate new growth

Let's start with this one:

This formula stimulates hair growth it involves dairy products which is an added benefit because of the lactic and alpha-hydroxyl acids which also acts as an exfoliate.

3 Tablespoons Fenugreek seeds
2-4oz Greek Yogurt (you judge to make a paste)

Start by grinding the seeds into a powder and to the Greek yogurt let it sit for 30 minutes, it should have the consistency of a paste. After 30 minutes apply all over the scalp let sit without heat covered with a plastic cap and cotton around the base of the plastic cap, after 30 minutes, scrub treatment into scalp like a shampoo. Rinse well then follow the **RXHSW®** cleansing process.

Cypress & Gingko Scalp Treatment

Use a 4 oz dark amber bottle
2 oz. Safflower Oil
1 oz. Basix™* Oil
1% Cypress EO.
1% Gingko Herb

Warm oil up to 90°F in a prep bowl add Gingko to the Oils. Let cool lower than 40°F, add EO Let product sit overnight, strain the Gingko off add to 4oz bottle then apply to scalp leave-in do not wash out. This is a week to 2-week long treatment. Label the bottle with ingredients and date can be used for up to 6 months before turning rancid. (spoil)

Herbal Rinses

The following herbs can be steeped in boiling water or Apple Cider Vinegar, strained, then cooled to room temperature to create an herbal rinse for the treatment of hair loss. Great for client experiencing visual signs of thinning or hair loss.

Basil Rinse

Apple Cider Vinegar

1 tsp. Basil

1 tsp. Rosemary

1 tsp. Sage

Warm Apple Cider Vinegar do not boil! Place Fresh Herbs in Vinegar for 1-2 weeks. Strain vinegar from herbs, Rinse is ready for use.

Vinegar Rinse:

1 c. Apple Cider Vinegar

5 dr. EO of your choice for anti-fungal use

Warm Apple Cider Vinegar do not boil! Place Fresh Herbs in Vinegar for 1-2 weeks. Strain vinegar from herbs, Rinse is ready for use.

For Shiny Hair & Healthy Scalp

2 c. Distilled Water

3 stalks of Fresh Rosemary Herb

1 Tbsp. Coconut Oil

Boil water for five min. Remove pot add water to sealable glass/plastic container add Rosemary and coconut Oil. Let sit for 1-2 days. Use as a leave-in or as a treatment after shampoo/cleaner. **Do not Rinse out.**

Hair Gloss

Grapeseed Oil

Coconut Oil

Massage your created blend into your scalp for daily use. For best use warm the oils to 80°F. Not higher, apply the oils to the scalps wrap hair with warm moist (place moist in towel in microwave for a minute at time until it warm enough for you) this type of treatment opens up the pores for maximum absorption of the treatment. You can also apply this before bed, strongly suggest a hair scarf to protect the bedding, remember these are oil based products. EOs can also be added to current shampoos and conditioners for at home regimens. Thus turning the shampoo into an herbal base shampoo

Hair Loss Remedies Treatments

Use a 4oz dark amber bottle

2-ounce RXHSW® Basix Oil *(this oil has every necessary ingredient for hair skin and nails) may be purchased via Rxestoratives.com website. For proven results follow formulas as written*

1-ounce Carrier Oil (Jojoba Oil or Grapeseed Oil, or Coconut Oil)

4 drops Spearmint E. O.

4 drops Orange E. O.

4 drops Grapefruit E. O.

4 drops Sage E. O.

4 drops Sea Kelp Extract

4 drops Burdock Root Extract

Warm Carrier Oil to 90° F. Let Cool for ten minutes add E. O.. Apply to scalp massage in leave in. Its best to do this treatment on the weekend to leave in overnight or all weekend. First complete the RX® Shampoo Method **RXHSW®** on page 182.

Hair Loss Oil

This formula takes 2 weeks to mature

2 oz. Sweet Almond Oil or Carrier oil of your choice

1tsp. Horsetail Fresh herbs

1tsp. Coltsfoot Fresh herbs

1tsp. Nettle Fresh herbs

May add four dr. E. O. of your choice use Stimulant E. O.

Warm the oil to 120 F°. Add herbs to oil while cooling. Leave herbs in oil. Pour into a tight sealed jar keep sealed for 2 weeks. Strain oil off of herbs use product at will.

❖ **To Sooth and Refresh the Scalp**

Use a 4oz. Dark amber Bottle

1-ounce RXHSW® Basix Oil *(this oil has every necessary ingredient for hair skin and nails) may be purchased via Rxestoratives.com website. For proven results follow formulas as written*
1-ounce Carrier oil *(choose the oil that's best for your hair use one of the carrier oil of your choice based on your issue*)

- 2 drops Tea tree
- 2 drops Lavender
- 2 drops Clary sage
- 2 drops Spearmint

Relax Sooth Stimulate Scalp

Use a 4oz. Dark amber Bottle

1-ounce RXHSW® Basix Oil *(this oil has every necessary ingredient for hair skin and nails) may be purchased via Rxestoratives.com website. For proven results follow formulas as written*
1-ounce (Jojoba or Sweet Almond)

- 1/2 ounce of base oil
- 2 drops Roman chamomile
- 2 drops Lavender
- 2 drops Sandalwood

- 2 drops Basil
- 1 drop Black Pepper

For Damaged, dry itchy scalp oil

I used a large 4-6 oz. amber colored bottle with a lotion pump attachment and added the following EOs:

3 oz Carrier Oil of choice (find the carrier oil best for you)

50 drops of Rosemary
40 drops of Lavender
20 drops of Sage
20 drops of Carrot Seed
10 drops of Helichrysum

Excellent for scalp problems like dandruff and itchy scalp

❖ **Natural Castile Shampoo**

Formula:

- 1 cup Pure Castile Soap
- ½ cup Witch Hazel
- 1 teaspoon Chamomile Oil
- 1 teaspoon Rosemary
- 1 teaspoon other EO for dandruff. Find the EO of your choice for dandruff

  Remember to write down the formula and label the bottle for future references.

Double boiler pot warm Castile Soap in pot. Bring to 70°F.

Reduce heat cool Soap to 50° F add Witch Hazel and E. O. Stir gently until thoroughly blended.

Pour the mixture into a squeezable bottle.

Apply to scalp after conditioner remember the RXHSW® Cleansing method.

Then style hair as usual

❖ ***Energizing Blend Shampoo:***

This Blends improves blood circulation to the scalp, leaving you awake and refreshed. Improving circulation has been known to slow down hair loss.

Ingredients:

- 2 oz. (30 ml) Liquid Castile Soap may be purchased at health food stores
- 3 drops Grapefruit EOs*
- 3 drops Peppermint EOs*
- 3 drops Spearmint*
- 2 drops Lavender EOs *

❖ ***Jojoba Hair Conditioner***

This conditioner will make hair smoother, softer and easy to manage.

Ingredients:

- 1 cup Rose Water
- 1 tablespoon jojoba oil
- 10 drops vitamin E oil

Instructions:

Warm the rose floral water with double boiler and add jojoba oil plus vitamin E. Blend the mixture with blender and do it at high speed for two mins

To use:

- Rinse the hair, then apply treatment add a little of treatment in your shampoo and conditioner for a full treatment.
- Leave the conditioner on with the treatment in it for a while (20-30 minutes) if you have damaged hair but if you don't, rinse after 15 minutes
- Put small amount of shampoo and do it lightly, wash hair it with cool water.

Treat dandruff with light, fragrance-free conditioners. Dandruff is a scalp issue, not a hair issue; the skin on your scalp grows and dies at a faster rate than in people without dandruff, leaving an embarrassing flaky white residue in your hair and on your shoulders. The shampoo you choose will have more of an effect on your dandruff than your conditioner, but there are still many products on the market geared toward treating this condition.

Look for lighter conditioners rather than high moisturizing or oil-heavy ones that can contribute to the problem on your scalp.[9]

Hair products with heavy fragrances often irritate the scalp, which leads to more itching, and more evidence of your dandruff on your clothes. Avoid heavily perfumed conditioners.

For dandruff, Massage oil into the scalp using your fingertips before going to bed and leave it on all night. You should cover every part of the scalp. Wash the hair in the morning. For best results, use sesame oil daily for 30 days.

❖ ***Dandruff- Tight Itchy Scalp and Prevention Blend:***

- 1 ounce Carrier Oil (Jojoba or Sesame Oil)
- 4 drops Spearmint
- 2 drops Basil
- 2 drops Lavender
- 2 drops Tea Tree
- 2 drops Rosemary
- 1 drop Ylang Ylang

To make formula concentrated double the EO drops per 1 oz Carrier Oil. Add formula to a 4 oz or 2 oz amber dropper bottle.

Remember to label all bottles, date and store them in a cool controlled place.

❖ *Anti-Dandruff Shampoo*

This is quite a strong blend which can be used to combat dandruff a dry scalp and itchy, flaky skin. Using a cupful of vinegar as a rinse with water this will improve the condition of scalp and help the hair.

Apple cider vinegar restore a natural pH to the skin and hair.

Directions: Leave Rinse on for 15 minutes Rinse well then follow up with the Leave-In-Conditioner* or the one you make yourself. Style as usual.

Ingredient:

Shampoo for dandruff

- 30 ml liquid castile soap
- 5 drops Lemon EOs
- 2 drops Rosemary EOs
- 3 drops Lavender EOs
- Vinegar Rinse:
    - 1 c. Apple Cider Vinegar
    - 5 dr. EO of your choice for anti-fungal use

❖ *Dandruff and Psoriasis Treatment*

- 2oz Castor Oil
- 1oz Sesame Oil
- 1oz Coconut Oil

- Mix oils together warm in a double boiler. Heat up 120° F, stir. Let cool then apply
- evenly all over hair. Place plastic cap over hair leave on for 30-45 minutes, Rinse with cool water, light conditioner, apply Oil based Leave-in Conditioner, for those with oily hair use citrus EO in Hot Oil Treatment.

❖ ***Treat Alopecia Dual Hair Growth Treatment***

Ylang Ylang E. O.*
Lavender E. O.*
Grapeseed Carrier Oil*
2 oz. Carrier Oil
4 drops Ylang Ylang
4 drops Lavender

Add E. O. to Carrier Oil in a dark Amber bottle. Store in a cool dry place for 24 hours before application to hair and scalp. evenly distribute oils place plastic cap with warm towels or a medium dry heat for 30 minutes. Rinse using the RXHSW process but NO SHAMPOO. Apply oil treatment sparingly three times week.

❖ ***Thicker Hair***

Purchase Rxestoratives Oil Blend: Basix*
Castor Oil*
Coconut Oil*
Avocado Butter*
Vitamin E

Melt Avocado butter in double boiler, add other oils warm for 15 minutes to allow the oils to blend together. Let product cool add natural preservative.

❖ **Nail Fungus**

2 oz Carrier Oil
5 gr Neem Oil
5 dr Tea Tree Oil
5 dr Rosemary
5 dr Basil E. O.

Warm carrier oil 120° F, add Neem Oil, let cool to 70° F add E. O.

Add oil to the fungus nail, then add formula to warm-hot water, dip nail(s) in the oil for 15-20 minutes pat the nails dry. Do Not Wash hands for 2 hours or more- best to do this treatment at night when going to sleep. This oil will stimulate healthy nail growth.

For Dandruff formula use apply to scalp after C.S.C. Let sit overnight or Leave-In…depending on mix it should smell great.

2 oz Castor Oil, Sesame, or Olive Oil

6 drops of your choice: Mix and match

Thyme

Clove

Eucalyptus
Tea Tree
Lavender should be used to off-set the fragrance

THE SKIN

Formula suggested Uses for Eczema

In a warm bath use E.O. to soak for hydrating Eczema and to control flare ups.

Carrier Oil:

Coconut Oil, Sweet Almond Oil Borage Seed Oil

12 drops of E.O. you can do 3 drops of one and 4 drops of another to equal 12 drops or just one E. O. to Equal 12 drops

Thyme	Clove
Eucalyptus	Bergamot
Chamomile	Tea Tree
Black Pepper	Lavender

To make a quick natural hydrating cream use, place shea butter in microwave for 30 seconds add E. O. let cool and use when necessary.

8 oz of Shea butter

20 drops of E. O. of choice (best use for this type of issue)

For an anti-itch, Mist for this type of issue. Mix ingredients in bottle shake well before each use, it will separate but that is ok..

4 oz Distilled Water

4 oz Carrier of choice (for this issue)

12 drops each;

Lavender

Tea Tree

Clove

Rosemary

Onion Juice

Onions are packed full of sulfur which stimulates the production of collagen in your skin. While you may initially cringe at the idea of applying onion juice to your scalp – or any of your skin for that matter – consider that it is one of the best natural remedies for combating hair loss. Lack of collagen in the hair is one of the biggest causes of thinning hair.

RXESTORATIVES PRODUCTS

HAIR PRODUCTS	USE	REGIMEN
CITRUS SODA	USE FIRST THEN MAKE A PASTE AND APPLY TO HAIR & SCALP LIKE YOUR FIRST SHAMPOO. FOLLOW THIS WITH A CONDITIONER	PERFORM THIS PROCESS THREE TIMES PER YEAR
MINT CONDITIONER	RXESTORATIVES STEP 1 & 3	ALWAYS USE CONDITIONER SHAMPOO & CONDITIONER WHEN WASHING THE HAIR
MINT SHAMPOO	RXESTORATIVES STEP 2. THIS STIMULATING SHAMPOO GREAT FOR HAIR GROWTH	DO NOT OVER USE THIS PRODUCT. MORE IS NOT BETTER. ONE SHAMPOO ONLY!

HAIR PRODUCTS	USE	REGIMEN
OILS OF NATURE	RXESTORATIVES PREMIUM OIL FOR HAIR GROWTH	USE 2-3 TIME PER WEEK. APPLY TO SCALP AND MASSAGE IN WELL
ACV30	RXESTORATIVES LEAVE-IN CONDITIONER THIS PRODUCT IS APPLE CIDER VINEGAR BASE THAT CONTINUALLY STIMULATES GROWTH	APPLY TO HAIR AFTER STEP 3 (1&3) THIS IS A LEAVE-IN DO NOT WASH OUT
BOARS BRUSH	USE DAILY BRUSH TO STIMULATE HAIR GROWTH.	THIS IS A NATURAL BRISTLE BRUSH

Q&A WITH PAMELA MAIR

Use the following "Personal Notes" pages to jot down your learnings, observations and notes for making your healthy hair at home a reality.

Q. My daughter is 12 and her hair is falling out, at 12! There are strands of hair in the bathroom on the floor everywhere.

A This sounds like she has entered in puberty and her hormonal levels in her body are changing. The hair loss will accelerate during this process and will slow down and even stop once her hormone levels are balanced off. If you as the parent feel that this is excessive hair loss go to her pediatrician and get a blood test done for an evaluation of vitamin deficiencies the main ones to pay attention to are Vitamin B12, Folic and Iron. When these vitamins a low this could contribute to hair loss.

Q. Are there medications that cause hair loss?

A. When you are dealing with high blood pressure, high cholesterol, any type of allergies even depression and are taking medication for any disorder you may have this may contribute to hair loss. It would be best to follow up with you doctor about any concerns you have about the medication they have prescribed for you. Do some research yourself to learn about the side effects.

Q. Does shampooing your hair (shampoo & conditioner) to often lead to hair loss?

A. Anything in excess will lead to an unfavorable consequence. In this case to answer the question, Yes. Due to the ingredients used in products excessive washing conditioning even "hair treatments" will lead to thinning, weakening of the tresses (strands). Do everything in moderation for best results. Remember to follow the product label instructions.

Q. I changed hairdressers and as soon as I started going to this new hairdresser, my hair began to fall out. Do you think it's because I changed hairdressers?

A. This is a twofold question:

1. If your hair was falling out before you left this answers your question. However;
2. If your hair begins to fall out after a week or two of going to the new stylist/hairdresser then two things:

a) Breakage does not start within one to two week of seeing a new stylist/hairdresser. It takes at least 4-6 weeks before you will even notice the hair is falling out or thinning. Weeks after a "Bad" relaxer or an over processed hair chemical service is when you notice that something is not right. If you had a perm/relaxer and changed stylist a week or two after this chemical service, then this was not the new stylist/hairdresser fault sorry it was your last stylist/hairdresser's fault. This was a problem/issue long before now, it was just never addressed. In this case, the client should apologize to the present hair stylist. □

b) If at any time after leaving the old stylist/hairdresser you experienced a serious shock(trauma) of information, had a car accident, lifestyle change (divorce), was fired from your job, death in the family, had surgery of any type big or small, major or minor (dentist) surgery this would contribute to hair loss as well. Or maybe your hormone balance is out of wack. See your doctor about this.

Q. What are the best vitamins for hair growth? Currently, I am taking fish oil, vitamin B-16, a multivitamin, calcium, vitamin E, and an amino acid supplement. So far this has helped my hair significantly. Any suggestions on vitamins to take for hair growth?

A. Omega 3•6•9 if you are not allergic to seafood/shellfish, Liquid Silica, Biotin with Magnesium and Vitamin E.

Q. Vitamin E for hair growth. Which would give me maximal results, consuming it or apply it directly to the hair? I hear that Vitamin E has great beneficial hair growth but I do not know how to use it. Are the capsules, the oil, or which is best to take? Please help.

A. In the Dosage section of this book you will find the appropriate suggested dosage of use. Follow the directions on the vitamin packaging for best results. To answer the question Vitamin E is good with an additional suggestion of Liquid Silica.

Q. What works best for hair growth? Biotin, sea kelp, E-vitamin, carrot oil, or anything else?

A. All the above are excellent vitamins, minerals for hair care.

Personal Note Page

Personal Note Page

Personal Note Page

Personal Note Page

Personal Note Page

Personal Note Page

Personal Note Page

Personal Note Page

Personal Note Page

Personal Note Page

Personal Note Page

Personal Note Page

Personal Note Page

Personal Note Page

Table of Abbreviations

Abbriviation	**Definition**
A	Avoid
A	Answer
ACV	Apple Cidar Vinegar
B	Beneficial
C	Cup
Dr	Drop
EO	Essential Oil
F	Fehrenheidt
LG	Large
N	Neutral
NB	Neutral / Beneficial
O	Occassional
OZ	Ounce
Q	Question
R	Rare
Tsp	Tablespoon
tsp	Teaspoon

INGREDIENTS GLOSSARY

-A-

ACACIA GUM: A soothing mucilage, thickener and stabilizer.

ACEROLA BERRY: Rich in sugars, minerals & flavonoids. A powerful source of vitamin C that helps stimulate connective tissue formation and the collagen-elastin network.

ACETONE: solvent commonly used in fingernail polish removers and toners; can be drying and irritating depending on concentration.

ACETIC ACID: Occurs naturally in apples, grapes, oranges, skimmed milk and a variety of other fruits and plants. It has disinfecting properties

ACETYLATED LANOLIN ALCOHOL: An alcohol that is not drying. Helps soften skin; is highly comedogenic (causes blackheads and/or whiteheads).

ALCOHOL SD-40: sometimes listed as SD Alcohol 40 and alcohol SDA-40, it is a high grade purified cosmetic alcohol. Evaporates instantly, so it is used as a vehicle to transport important ingredients to the skin's surface and then leave them there; gentler to the skin than ethyl (rubbing) alcohol. May help kill bacteria.

ALGAE/Seaweed Extract: an emollient, restoring moisture content to skin; claims to have antioxidant properties.

ALLANTOIN: a botanical thought to have skin calming properties; possibly reduces irritation.

ALPHA HYDROXY ACID: Considered an active ingredient that comes from the acids of fruit. This ingredient exfoliates the epidermis, the top layer. It also encourages moisture restoration and assist in helping other ingredients absorb into the skin. This is a hallmark ingredient for anti-aging and skin bleaching products. But beware of the sun it make the skin very sensitive to it.

ALPHA LIPOIC ACID: an antioxidant; is both water and fat soluble so it can protect many areas of a cell. Also, has anti-inflammatory properties.

ALUM: usually in crystal or powder form; has strong astringent properties; used in stypic sticks, popular with men who often nick themselves shaving.

AMINO ACIDS: The building blocks of protein. Some amino acids (essential amino acids) are not produced in the body and must be supplied externally. They are necessary for the hair, skin, nail and connective tissue growth.

AMODIMETHICONE: A form of silicone oil, it is an emollient and moisturizer, and provides silkiness. It is well tolerated by even the most sensitive skins.

AMPHOTERIC SURFACTANTS: Those in which the active molecule bears both positive and negative charges. Their properties depend upon th pH of the system and they may behave like anionic or cationic. Some of the finest amphoteric are used in shampoo systems formulated for dry or chemically treated hair due to their mildness and light conditioning properties.

AMMONIUM LAURYL SULFATE: The ammonium salt of lauryl sulfate derived from the natural coconut alcohols, it is a mild anionic surfactant widely used at acidic (mild) pH values.

ANTIMOCROBIAL: Ingredients that kill microorganisms, or prevent or inhibit their growth and reproduction.

ANTIOXIDANT: Ingredients that prevent or slow deterioration due to chemical reaction with oxygen.

ANGELICA: (Angelica archangelica). An herb with bactericidal and fungicidal properties, it is also calming to the skin

AONORI: A green algae containing large amounts of sulfated polysaccharides providing water-retaining properties for deep tissue moisture.

APPLES: Rich in natural pectin, containing polysaccharides, vitamin B, flavonoids and a high level of " malic" acid. This acid has been scientifically proven to be one of the 5 most beneficial AHAs that help stimulate and speed skin cell renewal. The other acids are "glycolic", from the heart of the raw cane sugar plant, "citric", from citrus fruit, "lactic" from milk, and "tartaric" from fruit fermentation, similar to that found in wine sediment. **Astringent; smoothes and tightens. Contains zinc.**

APPLE CIDER: Detoxifying. When added to a toner's formulation it acts as an "acid rinse" to adjust the skin's own pH.

APRICOT EXTRACT: Rich in vitamin A, beta-carotene and zinc, it has softening, cleansing, and soothing properties.

ARYLATES COPOLYMER: active ingredient in an oil-absorbing gel, such as Clinac O.C.

ASCORBIC ACID: vitamin C; an antioxidant and stimulant of collagen synthesis by skin cells (fibroblasts). Can also have skin lightening effect in certain preparations. Only L-ascorbic acid (as opposed to D-ascorbic acid) is effective.

ASCORBYL PALMITATE: fat-soluble vitamin C derivative. Good antioxidant but less effective than vitamin C for stimulating collagen synthesis.

AVOCADO OIL: Natural oil rich in vitamins and minerals. It is an excellent skin conditioner and moisturizer that readily penetrates the skin.

AZULENE: An essential oil derived from the German chamomile flower (matricaria chamomilla). It is an excellent analgesic, detoxifier, and anti-inflammatory, and extremely soothing and calming to the skin.

-B-

BAKING SODA: Sodium bicarbonate. Adjust pH, stabilizes viscosity. Aids in cleansing oily skin.

BANANA EXTRACT: Contains vitamins A, B, and F. It softens, and smooths the skin.

BARLEY: A demulcent. Soothing. Combined with tomato, it helps improve penetration, creating a delivery system to suspend the critical components and facilitate delivery into the stratum corneum, the outermost layer of the epidermis consisting of dead cells that slough off.

BASIL: The sweet energizing aroma of basil is good for fatigue and is an excellent mental tonic. When blended with other oils it is restorative and balancing. Oily hair. Promotes growth Adds moisture and prevents split ends

BEE PROPOLIS: Tree resin collected by bees to line their hives; it is antiseptic and possibly anti-biotic.

BEESWAX: Obtained from the honeycomb of the honeybee. Used as an emulsifier, thickener, it is a sticky wax like ingredient found in many cosmetic products. It provides moisture and acts as a wall between water and oil it allows them to blend together. May tend to cause blackhead and possibly block pores. This is a natural derived emulsifier and thickener.

BEHENALCONIUM CHLORIDE: see Quaternary Ammonium Salts. Used in many hair conditioners and rinses.

BENTONITE: Natural clay from volcanic ash. Used in facial masks for it's drawing abilities.

BENZETHONIUM CHLORIDE: A detergent type ammonium found in hair products. It's a preservative that aids in broad spectrum of microorganisms like: (fungi, bacteria, algae). Normally used in concentrations less than 0.5%. This ingredient is found in other hair & skin cosmetics. It is also an antibacterial and is highly toxic.

BENZOPHENONE-3 (oxybenzone), Benzophenone-4 (sulisobenzone) Blocks UV radiation in sunscreen.

BENZOYL PEROXIDE: antibacterial agent that kills acnes, the germ responsible for acne breakouts. Can be drying and/or irritating. Some develop high skin sensitivity to benzoyl peroxide.
Available in both prescription and OTC forms ranging from 2.5 to 10%.

BENZYL ALCOHOL: Antibacterial preservative typically used in concentrations 1 to 3%. May cause skin irritation.

BERGAMOT: Most people know this aroma through Earl Grey tea, which is flavored with bergamot oil. It is a fruity citrus oil of spicy-floral freshness. Bergamot is excellent for uplifting moods and is especially helpful in relieving anxiety, stress, tension and depression. herb, antiseptic, anti-inflammatory properties, aromatic, skin balancer, useful for treatment of acne, soothing, stress reducer, calm irritated skin, psoriasis and stress.

BETA HYDROXY ACID: a subclass of organic acids; the most common one is salicylic acid, a long term ingredient used for exfoliation of dry skin as well as for acne therapy.

BETA CAROTENE: Found in all plant and many animal tissues, used as coloring in cosmetics. Used also as antioxidant. Precursor of Vitamin A occurring naturally in plants, especially abundant in carrots, papaya and algae. It possesses both healing and cellular renewal properties. A natural emulsifier and thickener.

BHT: Potent synthetic oil-soluble antioxidant often used as a preservative against rancidity.

BIOTIN: A naturally occurring vitamin H. One of the B complex vitamins used to improve the texture of creams and add body and shine to hair products. Some studies show that it has a positive effect on hair growth when taken internally.

BISABALOL: Chamomile oil. Moisturizing, soothing and anti-inflammatory

BLUE GREEN ALGAE: The smallest and most primitive of plants that contain chlorophyll in their protoplasm. Their unicellular bodies contain all the biological constituents necessary for life functions. Hydrates and protects skin.

BLUE MALLOW: Cleansing, non-irritating, and softening.

BUTTER: Any of various fatty oils remaining nearly solid at room temperature.

BUTYLENE GLYCOL: Organic humectant similar to propylene glycol.

BUTYL PARABEN: A member of the paraben family of petrochemicals commonly used as a preservative to prevent mold, fungus, and bacteria.

-C-

CALENDULA: (Marigold) Astringent, cleansing, anti-inflammatory, moisturizing, soothing, softening and an anti-oxidant.

CARRAGEEN: A gel-forming polysaccharide found in the "red algae" seaweed known as "Irish moss". Soothing, and a natural emulsifier.

CAMPHOR: a cooling agent; may help alleviate the symptoms of itching and irritation.

CARBOMERS (934, 940, 941, 980, 981): stabilizers and thickeners common in skin care products.

CARROT JUICE: High in both alpha & beta-carotenoids (possibly more powerful than beta carotene alone) which are responsible for Pro-vitamin A activity in formulation. Soothing and healing.

CARROT SEED OIL: An essential oil used in formulation to help quiet dermatitis, eczema, psoriasis, and rashes. It's high content of Vitamins A, C, B and B2 relieves dryness in mature skin.

CASTOR OIL: A natural emollient which gives body and shine to the hair and helps restore a natural, healthy appearance. It is very useful for skin and hair related complaints like rashes, eczema, dry hair. A superb conditioner that has been proven to strengthen the hair shaft. for beautiful eyebrows and eyelashes. Applying pure

castor oil to your eyebrows and lashes, particularly those who have scanty growth will make them grow thick and long. It is used in lipsticks, concealers, hair pomade, ointments, creams and lotions. Acts as a humectant with soothing and emollient actions. Boosts lather in handcrafted soaps.

CAFFIENE: used to alleviate puffiness under eyes.

CALENDULA: (Marigold) Astringent, cleansing, anti-inflammatory, moisturizing, soothing, softening and an anti-oxidant.

CHAMOMILE: Healing, extremely soothing, and moisturizing.

CARRAGEEN: A gel-forming polysaccharide found in the "red algae" seaweed known as "Irish moss". Soothing, and a natural emulsifier.

CARROT JUICE: High in both alpha & beta-carotenoids (possibly more powerful than beta carotene alone) which are responsible for Pro-vitamin A activity in formulation. Soothing and healing.

CARROT SEED OIL: An essential oil used in formulation to help quiet dermatitis, eczema, psoriasis, and rashes. It's high content of Vitamins A, C, B and B2 relieves dryness in mature skin.

CETALKONIUM CHLORIDE: This ingredient is in the ammonium family. Its an antibacterial ingredient .

CERAMIDES: A very scarce and costly ingredient also is a epidermal hydrating agent.

CETEARETH: Is an alcohol, combined ceteary together stearyl used as a lubricant.

CELLULOSE: polymer from plant cell walls; used as a thickener and emulsifier.

CETRIMONIUM CHLORIDE: Quaternary conditioning agent, similar to cetrimonium bromide, but more suitable for water systems.

CETYL ALOCHOL: Lubricant and emulsifier. Nonirritating, nondrying, non-comedogenic.

CETYLDIMONIUM CHLORIDE: Used often as a conditioning agent, compatible with surfactants, often used in shampoos.

CHAMOMILE: Healing, extremely soothing, and moisturizing. Herbal therapy for conditioning

CITRIC ACID: A natural, edible organic acid used to adjust pH, Found in plants and citrus fruits. This organic acid is a pH adjuster and acts as a preservative and anti-oxidant, one of the natural hydroxy acids derived from citrus fruits.

CHLOROPHYLL: The green component of plants that has antiseptic and anti-fungal properties

CHLOROXYLENOL: A crystalline, water soluble substance used as an antiseptic, germicide and fungicide. Penetrates skin. No known toxicity in humans when diluted below 20%.

CLARY SAGE: All types of hair. Dandruff treatment

CLOVE: Clove has valuable first aid benefits, specifically in dentistry as a pain killer. It is revitalizing and comforting. The oil should not be used directly on the skin

COCOA BUTTER: Vegetable fat solid at room temperature but liquid at body temperature. Due to this property often used in lip balms and massage creams. Considered comedogenic and may also (rarely) cause allergy.

COCONUT OIL: Coconut oil is hair conditioner. This highly saturated fat is commonly used to promote lather in soaps and gel. Wonderfully emollient and has cooling properties. It is emollient on skin and hair.

CO-ENZYME Q 10: A natural substance found in every cell of the human body. It begins to decrease in the mid 20's. It comes from plants in their tissue. Co-enzyme Q 10 (also known as "ubiquinone") is a vitamin-like anti-oxidant that boosts cellular activity. It helps to fortify the skin's defenses against UV damage, plus reduce the appearance of wrinkles, strengthening cell membranes, and providing the skin with new energy.

COCAMIDE DEA/MEA/MIPA – Synthetic non-ionic surfactants. These and other surfactants beginning with 'coco –' or 'coca –' are referred to as 'natural' and 'derived from coconut oil'. They are not natural and coconut oil is used for synthesizing great many chemical compounds, as are many other natural oils.

COLLAGEN: the main supporting fiber located within the dermis, gives strength and provides structure. You cannot replace lost collagen by simply applying it to your skin due to its large molecule size. However, topical collagen can act as a moisturizing agent.

COLTSFOOT: Soothing, and healing, which is a superb skin nutrient. A healing herb with soothing and softening (emollient) properties.

CYCLIC ACID: a new term for Hyaluronic Acid, an effective humectant/moisturizing agent.

COMFREY: One of the most famed healing plants; it contains allantoin, a substance that promotes the growth of connective tissue and is easily absorbed through the skin. Moisturizing, rejuvenating!

CONEFLOWER: (Echinacea) Anti-inflammatory, soothing to skin and scalp.

CORNSTARCH: Starch obtained from corn and used as an oil absorbent in cosmetics

CUCUMBER: An anti-inflammatory. It has an extremely soothing effect on the skin.

CYCLOMETHICONE: form of silicone; gives products a smooth texture; noncomedogenic.

-D-

DEA (diethanolamine) : **DEA (diethanolamine), MEA (monoethanolamine), TEA (triethanolamine):** These toxins are used as emulsifiers or foaming agents. When they are combined with other chemicals they form cancer causing nitrates and nitrosamines. They are **hormone disrupting chemicals**. The National Toxicology Program (NTP), found in 1998, an association between the topical application of DEA and certain DEA–related ingredients and cancer in lab animals. These chemicals cause allergic reactions, are eye irritants and cause excessive drying of the hair and skin. These chemicals are restricted in Europe due to known carcinogenic effects. Samuel Epstein, Professor of Environmental Health at the University of Illinois, reports that repeated skin applications of DEA based detergents resulted in a major increase in the incidence of Liver and Kidney Cancer.

DEA will be listed in the following ways: **Cocamide DEA, Cocamide MEA, DEA–Cetyl Phosphate, DEA–Oleath–3 Phosphate, Larramide DEA, Linoleamide MEA, Myristamide DEA, Oleamide DEA, Stearamide MEA, TEA–Luryl Sulfate, Triethanolamine.**

DECYL -POLYGLUCOSE: Vegetable based surfactant.

DEIONIZED WATER: Water purified by deionization technique based on removal of highly active ions especially positively charged cations like calcium (Ca++) magnesium(MG++) and iron (Fe++) and (Fe+++).

DIMETHICONE: a form of silicone; skin protectant; moisture sealant; noncomedogenic; has been used in some scar therapies.

DMDM (Hydantonin) and Urea (Imidazolidinyl), Diazolidinyl Urea: Commonly used preservatives *(trade name **Germall 115**)* that release formaldehyde. These chemicals cause skin irritation
(American Academy of Dermatology) as well as irritation to the respiratory system. In many it can cause skin allergies (contact dermatitis), headache, chest pain, dizziness and depression. Material Safety Data Sheets (MSDS) list the toxicology of these chemical substances as harmful by inhalation, ingestion and through skin absorption. This toxin is 17.7% formaldehyde.

DRY MILK: Like liquid milk it contains "natural" lactic acid. (Moisturizing properties).

DULSE: A flat leaved red sea weed ("Fucus"). It is high in bio-nutritional vitamins including B1, B2, B3, B5, B6, B9 and Beta-carotene. It stimulates connective tissue repair and is cell energizing.

-E-

EDTA: preservative; slows down degradation (e.g. oxidation) of ingredients by chelating (grabbing and shielding) catalytic trace metals; may cause contact dermatitis.

ELLAGIC ACID: Ellagic acid is a compound found in raspberries, strawberries, cranberries, walnuts, pecans, pomegranates, and other plant foods. A super antioxidant. **Guar**

EMULSIFYING WAX: Vegetable waxes that are treated so that they mix more easily with other ingredients.

ENZYMES: Protein that act as a catalyst in some chemical reactions.

EVENING PRIMROSE OIL: Calming, cleansing, and moisturizing. High in essential fatty acids; especially gamma-linolenic acid.

EYEBRIGHT: Astringent, cleansing.

EMOLLIENT: Ingredients that act as lubricants on the skin surface, which give the skin a soft and smooth appearance.

EMULSION: A mixture of two liquids that normally cannot be mixed, in which one liquid is dispersed in the other liquid as very fine droplets. Emulsifying agents are often used to help form the emulsion and stabilizing agents are used to keep the resulting emulsion from separating. The most common emulsions are oil-in-water emulsions (where oil droplets are dispersed in water) and water-in-oil emulsions (where water droplets are dispersed in oil).

EMULSIFYING WAX: Vegetable waxes that are treated so that they mix more easily with other ingredients. - Used to combine oils with water when manufacturing lotions and creams.

ENZYMES: Protein that act as a catalyst in some chemical reactions.

ESSENTIAL OIL: A concentrated liquid containing volatile aroma compounds from plants.

ESTER: An organic compound formed by the reaction of an acid with an alcohol.

EXFOLIANT: Ingredients that help to remove dead skin cells from the skin surface.

EUCALYPTUS: Eucalyptus is a traditional household remedy that has strong antiseptic and decongestant properties that is often used in saunas and vapor rubs. It is refreshing, opening and purifying.

EVENING PRIMROSE OIL: Calming, cleansing, and moisturizing. High in essential fatty acids; especially gamma-linolenic acid. Rich source of GLA.

EYEBRIGHT: Astringent, cleansing.

-F-

FATTY ACIDS: Natural organic compound that consists of a carboxyl group (oxygen, carbon and hydrogen). Animal and vegetable fats are made up of various combinations of fatty acids (in sets of three) connected to a glycerol molecule, making them triglycerides. (Essential Fatty Acids or Vitamin F) Necessary for regulating healthy skin. Helps prevent premature aging.

FENNEL: Cleansing, anti-bacterial, rejuvenating

FRAGRANCE: Substances that impart an odor to a product.

-G-

GERANIUM: Astringent, cleansing, moistening, softening, stimulating.

GLYCERYL MONSTEARATE: An emollient, emulsifier derived from natural stearic acid and glycerine.

GINGER: Purges and stimulates.

GLYCERIDES: Any class used as a texturizer and/ or emollient.

GLYCERIN: A humectant (water-attracting/binding ingredient), emulsifier, and emollient.

GLYCERYL STEARATE: Emulsifier and humectant. Produced from fatty acids and glycerin. Readily penetrates the skin.

GLYCOSAMINOGLYCANS: Found in all plants. Sodium hyaluronate and other glycosaminoglucans are vital moisturizers and lubricants present in the interstitial spaces between epidermal cells. The absence of these lubricating moisturizers can accelerate the deterioration of the skin's collagen, resulting in the loss of elasticity, flexibility and tonicity. They are conditioning, moisturizing, and promote suppleness & firmness.

GLYCOLIC ACID: Exfoliant, used in a wide range of exfoliating products, from exfoliating lotions to chemical peels. May improve fine lines. Overuse can cause skin irritation and other skin damage.

Glycol Stearate: Thickening agent that helps give products a luminescent or opalescent appearance.

GRAPES: Powerful free radical scavenger/anti-oxidant rich in sugars, minerals, flavonoids, vitamins in B group. Promotes cellular health rejuvenation. Percentage of AHAs: 10 citric, 5 malic, 10 tartaric.

GRAPEFRUIT: Stimulating, astringent, cleansing, exfoliating...anti-viral, a free-radical invader. Percentage of AHAs: 15 citric, 2.5 glycolic, 2.50 malic, 5 lactic. Benificial for oily type hair and skin.

GRAPEFRUIT SEED EXTRACT: a natural preservative that is a good substitute for the parabens, but more expensive.

GRAPE SEED OIL: Ultra fine oil with especially non-allergenic properties. Free-radical scavenger.

GREEN PAPAYA: It is an excellent free-radical scavenger and cellular renewal ingredient with the ability to digest protein, selecting only dead cells without harming the living ones. Green or un-ripened fruit contains the highest content of "papain". As the fruit matures this powerful enzyme decreases.

GUAR GUM: A natural resin from the seeds of an Asian tree. Thickener, plasticizer, and emulsifier.

GUAVA: Soothing and moisturizing, guava also contains vitamins A and C, beta-carotene and zinc.

GUM: substances exuded by plants that are gelatinous when moist but harden on drying. See http://www.cosmeticsinfo.org/glossary/letter_g#sthash.EEIEAkLc.dpuf

GREEN TEA EXTRACT: a botanical extract shown to be an effective antioxidant

GUAR GUM: Plant derived polysaccharide used as a thickening agent in skin care formulations.

-H-

HAIR FIXATIVE: Ingredients that help hair hold its style by inhibiting the hair's ability to absorb moisture.

HAIR STRAIGHTENING INGREDIENT/AGENT: Substances that modify hair fibers to facilitate changes to the structure of the fibers, such as with permanent waves or with hair straightening.

HAMAMELIS WATER: *(Witch hazel)* an astringent herb that possesses the ability to soothe the skin.

HONEY: A natural skin softener used in formulation as an emollient, humectants! Honey is anti-fungal and anti-bacterial, suggesting that it contains anti-microbial ingredients. It offers high levels of hydrogen peroxide. Peroxide stimulates white blood cells that initiate the body's immune response to infection. Honey contains other significant amounts of vitamins, including vitamin C and trace amounts of iron, copper, manganese, calcium, potassium, sodium, phosphorus and magnesium, all possibly adding to Honey's wound healing effect.

HORSETAIL - Rich in minerals the body uses to maintain healthy tissue. It facilitates the absorption of calcium by the body, which nourishes nails, skin, hair, bones, and the body's connective tissue. The herb helps eliminate excess oil from skin and hair. Help to regrow hair

HUMECTANT: Ingredients that slow the loss of moisture from a product during use and that increase the water content of the top layers of the skin by drawing moisture from the surrounding air

HORSETAIL - Rich in minerals the body uses to maintain healthy tissue. It facilitates the absorption of calcium by the body, which nourishes nails, skin, hair, bones, and the body's connective tissue. The herb helps eliminate excess oil from skin and hair. Help to regrow hair

HUMECTANT: Ingredients that slow the loss of moisture from a product during use and that increase the water content of the top layers of the skin by drawing moisture from the surrounding air.

HYALURONIC ACID: also referred to as a "cyclic acid"; an effective humectant/moisturizing agent.

HYDROQUINONE: skin pigmentation lightening agent; a maximum of 2% is sold over the counter; higher concentrations available by prescription.

HYDROLYZED HUMAN HAIR KERATIN PROTEIN: Protein derived from human hair by enzymatic/acidic hydrolyzation.

HYDRIXTETGEK CELLULOSE: Used as a thickener in creams and lotions.

HYDROXYPROPYLTRIMONIUM CHLORIDE - Naturally derived from Guar tree, cationic conditioning agent used frequently in shampoos.**Glycerin:** hydrates and provides a skin barrier against loss of moisure; allows topical agents to go on very smoothly; may clog pores when present in high concentrations.

May also increase moisture retention.

HYDROXYPROPYL Methylcellulose: Fibrous substance derived from the chief part of the cell walls of plants. Used as thickener and to give products uniform consistency and body.

-I-

IRISH MOSS: Brownish purple algae that grows attached to rocks at low tide marks. It is a rich source of the emollient and moisture binding substance carrageen, and many micro-nutrients

IRON OXIDE: A naturally occurring compound of iron and oxygen. Used as a natural colorant.

ISOSPROPYL ALCOHOL: vehicle with antibacterial properties; drying to the skin especially in higher concentrations.

ISOPROPYL PALMITATE: emollient usually derived from palm and/or coconut oil; may be comedogenic.

ISOSTEARIC ACID: Fatty acid that forms a film on the skin; may be comedogenic.

-J-

JASMINE: Moisturizing; calming to the skin.

JOJOBA OIL: natural wax not an oil. It is an effective emollient and lubricant and is an excellent oil for dandruff and helps promote hair growth.

-K-

KAOLIN (China Clay): used in oil-absorbing powders and masques; highly absorbent.

KOJIC ACID: skin lightener; sometimes promoted as a bleaching agent for ethnic skin.

-L-

LACTIC ACID- A natural, minor organic acid prepared by fermentation. One of the five most beneficial AHAs, it is naturally occurring in milk fermentation. A mild exfoliant that helps reduce wrinkles and improve the skin's texture. Sometimes found in blood, sour milk, sauerkraut, pickles, and other food products made by bacterial fermentation. Used in cosmetics to adjust acid/alkali balance. Lactic acid is a major factor in the skin's buffer system. Alpha hydroxy acid used in dermatology to hydrate and smooth dry, flaking skin. May occasionally be used in high concentrations as a chemical peel.

LACTOSE PEROXIDASE & GLUCOSE OXIDAISE: One part of this enzyme system is extracted from milk whey, the other is a naturally occurring nutritional carbohydrate sourced from microbial culture. These natural enzymes work together to prevent spoilage and bacterial growth in natural formulas

LAMINARIA DIGITATA: A giant kelp, rich in iodine and other trace elements and co-enzymes, make it valuable as a skin supplement for normalizing cellular function.

LANOLIN: emollient and moisturizer; obtained from sheep; a sensitizer like other wool derivatives, in eczema-prone individuals.

LAVENDER OIL: Astringent, calming, cleansing, moisturizing, softening, rejuvenating...and soothing with anti-bacterial properties. Normal hair. Scalp treatment for itchiness, dandruff, and even lice!

LECITHIN: emollient and emulsifier. From the Greek meaning "egg yolk". Natural antioxidant, emollient and emulsifier used in a variety of cosmetics. Egg yolk is 8 - 9% lecithin. A natural anti-oxidant and emollient mainly derived from common egg yolk or from naturally occurring phospholipids derived from soybeans. Helps protect the skin, soften the skin and replenish the acid mantle. Attracts water and acts as a moisturizer.

LEMON: Antibacterial, softening, anti-wrinkle, anti-oxidant, antiseptic. Percentage of AHAs: 15 citric, 2.5 glycolic, 2.5 malic, 5 lactic. Controls sebum and oily skin.

LEMON GRASS OIL: Distilled from the grassy herb of the same name; it purifies, and hydrates.

LEMON OIL: Expressed from the outer rind of the lemon, it acts as a mild bleach that can brighten dull skin and calm redness. Naturally astringent, antiseptic and bactericidal; abundant in vitamins A, B & C. Gives golden highlights; treatment for dry scalp, dandruff, lice, and underactive sebaceous glands

LICORICE EXTRACT: skin lightener; believed to be more potent than kojic acid.

LICORICE ROOT: Rebalances dermal cells & helps reduce the formation of melanin, (pigment that gives skin color); has significant healing effects on many skin diseases. Firming, soothing.

LIMNANTHIS ALBA OIL: From the seeds of the one year old Limnanthis Alba plants of Oregon. Its 97% fatty acid content and small molecule structure, make it one of the most penetrating oils available in skin care...and...it is one of the most stable lipids known.

LIME OIL: Antiseptic, bactericidal and restorative; high in vitamins A, B & C.

LINOLEIC ACID Essential fatty acid, emollient and emulsifier.

LIPID: Fat/ fat-like matter found in the cells of plants and animals that includes fats, waxes, oils, and related compounds.

LIPOSOMES: active ingredient delivery system; hollow spheres made from phospholipids (such as lecithin) that are up to 300 times smaller than skin cells. Liposomes are filled with active agents which they carry into the skin and then gradually release.

LYCOPENE: Abundant in the red flesh and skin of the tomato. It appears in very high concentration when tomatoes are processed...and is the most active carotenoid (one of nature's most important anti-oxidant families) in terms of anti-oxidant activity. It appears to strengthen cellular integrity and function. (Lycopene is one of the top 3 carotenoids found in human tissue and blood plasma). It is more than twice as powerful as beta-carotene at quenching free radicals.

LYSINE: Amino acid important for collagen production; possibly ineffectual topically for that purpose.

-M-

MAGNESIUM: A lightweight mineral occurring in nature. It is especially abundant in specific varieties of sea algae and salts from the sea. Magnesium can help re-mineralize and soothe the skin.

Magnesium Ascorbyl Phosphate: a vitamin C derivative; more stable than vitamin C; has comparable effectiveness as collagen synthesis booster.

MANDARIN OIL: Antiseptic, toning and bactericidal.

MANGANESE: A mineral occurring abundantly in mineral mud, sea salts and specific sea plants.

MENTHOL : It can be obtained naturally from peppermint and other mint oils. It cools the skin and is used in cosmetics, food and pharmaceutical industries. A local anesthetic. Nontoxic in low doses but if higher than 3% it can be irritating.

METHYL GLUCETH: a humectant/ moisturizing agent.

METHYLPARABEN: A preservative with anti-microbial abilities that prevents the formation of bacteria, and is effective in very low concentrations.

.

METHYLSULFONYYLMETHANE: (MSM) An organic bio-available form of sulfur, which is the "nuts and bolts" of the skin proteins. The sulfur bond is responsible for the strength, shape and resilience of the collagen, elastin, and keratin structures of the skin.

MICA: A transparent mineral that is mined from the earth. It can be opalescent, sparkling or completely matte. It is often treated with iron oxides to make brilliant colors and used in mineral powders for its' "slip" and light reflecting qualities.

MINERAL OIL, Parrafin, Petrolatum (Petro-Chemicals): These are derived from petroleum and coal. These chemicals coat the skin like plastic, clogging pores and decreasing the skin's ability to eliminate toxins. These toxins accumulate and can cause acne and other disorders of the skin. They also induce premature aging by slowing cellular development..

MUCOPOLYSACCHAILDES: safe and effective humectants.

MUGWORT: A stimulant. When combined in a complex with Algae, it has anti-stinging, anti-inflammatory and anti-irritant properties.

MUCOPOLYSACCARIDES: A gelatinous, basic component of the skin. Helps maintain a moist environment for collagen, elastin and dermal cells while providing support for connective tissue and mucous membranes. A humectant and skin softener.

MYRISTYL MYRISTATE: emollient; an ester of myristyl alcohol and myristic acid.

-N-

NAIL CONDITIONER AGENT: Ingredients that enhance the appearance and feel of nails, by moisturizing the nail, increasing nail sheen, or by reducing nail brittleness and flaking.

NANOSPHERES: active ingredient delivery system; micro-reservoir particles of porous polymers that have a special structure permitting high absorption and timed release of the agents into the skin.

NECTAR: Sweet liquid saccharine secreted by plant nectarines (glands); chief raw material of honey

NEEM:- From a plant found in India, neem oil is antibacterial, nourishing and helps the skin to retain moisture.

NETTLE: Derived from nuts and grains; heals, nourishes, increases scalp circulation and stimulates hair follicle**s.** Rich in minerals, purifies and tones. Can be used in hair preparations to aid in stimulating hair growth and improves the condition of the scalp. Rich in minerals and plant hormone**s.**

NONVOLATILES: The fraction of a substance that does not vaporize upon heating.

-O-

OAT BETA GLUCANS: A blend of oat extract and refined oat proteins. Together they form an invisible layer over the skin to help retain moisture while promoting the repair of skin cells. High levels of naturally occurring anti-oxidants help protect against cellular damage. Soothing, healing! OATS: Calming, cleansing, softening, and moisturizing.

OCTYL PALMITATE: nondrying, nongreasy solvent; often used in cleansers, astringents.

OLEIC ACID: A fatty acid occurring as a glyceride, triolein, in nearly all fats, and in many oils: olive, almond and cod-liver.

OLEORESIN: A natural plant product containing essential oil and resin.

OPACIFYING AGENT: Substances that reduce the clear or transparent appearance of cosmetic products. Some opacifying agents are used in skin make-up for hiding blemishes.

ORANGE OIL: (Sweet blossom). Astringent, bactericidal, moistening, softening and rejuvenating.

ORGANIC COMPOUND: A compound that contains carbon and hydrogen and usually other elements such as nitrogen, sulfur and oxygen.

OXIDIZING AGENT: Ingredients that restore hair or skin to its normal reacted state after exposure to a reducing agent in permanent waving, or the process that aid in oxidative hair dyeing.

-P-

PABA (Para-Aminobenzoic Acid): In the '70's sunscreens contained a 'UVB warning this ingredient can cause contact dermatitis.

PALMAROSA OIL: Brings exceptional hydration to the skin. Effectively renews skin cells.

PANTHENOL: A non-toxic, non-irritating vitamin B5, this plant-derived ingredient is added to skin care preparations where improved absorption of various nutrients is desirable. Research has shown that panthenol, a natural hydrator, penetrates into the lower skin layers where it is absorbed by skin cells and becomes pantothenic acid (Vitamin B5). As it penetrates to the deep layers of the skin, it helps diminish wrinkles by adding moisture under the skin. It is also a hair thickener and strengthener (plumping and moisturizing the hair shaft) that nourishes the scalp.

PAPAIN: Also known as **PAPAYA** This is an enzyme found in papaya, most potent from un-ripe green papaya. Dissolves dead skin cells

PARABENS: (Methylparaban-Ethylparaban-Propylparaban-Butylparaban-Isobutyl Paraban), also known as Alkyl parahydroxy benzoates: These are synthetic preservatives used in most personal care products. Parabans have been found to have hormone-disrupting qualities, such as the ability to mimic estrogen. Currently, this is of major concern to researchers since parabans have been found in breast cancer tissue. Parabens penetrate the skin and appear in the blood.

PATCHOULI: Oily hair. Dandruff treatment

PEACH: Rich in sugars, minerals (zinc), vitamins (vitamins A & C, beta carotene) and organic acids, particularly citric and malic. Moisturizing, soothing, toning, exfoliating. Percentage of AHAs: 10 citric, 5malic, 5 tartaric, 5 salicylic.

PECTIN: An enzyme extracted from citrus fruits and apples. Emulsifier, thickener, soothing.

PEG-60 Hydrogenated Castor Oil: A solvent and plasticizing agent that has been shown to cause cancer.

PEG 120 METHY GLUCOSE DIOLEATE: Conditioning agent from corn.

PEPPERMINT: Stimulating herb. Best for dry hair. Promotes hair growth.

PEPTIDE: A group of compounds made up of amino acid chains. An ingredient name containing the term peptide is usually synthetic.

pH- A measurement of the acidity or basicity of a substance. pH is the negative logarithm (base 10) of the concentration of hydrogen ions in solution. Water has a concentration of hydrogen ions of 1.0 x 10-7, and thus has a pH of 7. A pH of 7 is considered neutral, a pH lower than 7 is considered acidic, and a pH higher than 7 is considered basic.

pH ADJUSTER- Ingredients that are used to control the pH of cosmetic products.

PINEAPPLE JUICE: Contains abundance of the enzyme "bromelin" that dissolves dead skin cells. Has cleansing properties and serves as an antioxidant because of its active constituents: vitamin C, citric acid, and sugars. It is also a mild exfoliant, due to the presence of the enzyme bromelain.

PISTACHIO: Nut rich in calcium, thiamine, phosphorus, iron and vitamin A. Percentage of AHAs: 10 citric, 3.5 glycolic, 6 malic, 3.5 lactic, 2 tartaric.

PLANTAIN: Cell proliferating, astringent and healing.

POLYSORBATE 20: Derived from sorbitol. Used as a stabilizer. It has a soothing effect on the skin.

PROPYLPARABEN: Used as a preservative, bactericide and fungicide, it is effective against a large variety of contaminants at very low concentration.

PROTEIN: Necessary for all cellular functions. Protein is made up of complex combinations of amino acids and has a good similarity with the skin. They help retain water and reduce water loss on the skin's surface.

PETROLATUM: Heavy vehicle based on petroleum hydrocarbons, most commonly known for its use in Vaseline; good for sensitive skin but is occlusive and can cause or aggravate acne in susceptible individuals.

POLYBUTENE: helps make liquids texturally viscous.

POLY HYDROXY ACID: PHA, derived from the buds of fruit trees; is claimed to be gentler yet as effective as AHAs; still debatable.

POLYSORBATE 20: Derived from sorbitol. Used as a stabilizer. It has a soothing effect on the skin.

PRESERVATIVE: Ingredients that prevent or retard bacterial growth, and thus protect cosmetic products from spoilage.

PROLINE: amino acid vital to the composition and production collagen; possibly ineffective in topical products.

PROPYLPARABEN: Used as a preservative, bactericide and fungicide, it is effective against a large variety of contaminants at very low concentration.

PROPYLENE GLYCOL/Butylene Glycol (PG): This is used in personal care products as a moisture carrying ingredient. PG will strip the skin's natural barrier and is easily and rapidly absorbed, leaving the immune system vulnerable. The PG used by the cosmetics industry is also used by the automotive industry in the manufacture of anti–freeze and automotive brake fluid. In 1992, the FDA proposed a ban on propylene glycol. Propylene Glycol may also be listed as Butylene Glycol and Ethylene Glycol.PUMICE: Finely ground volcanic rock to cleanse and slough off dead skin.

PROTEIN: A naturally occurring complex organic substance present in relatively high amounts in meats, fish, eggs, cheese, legumes. Made of carbon, hydrogen, oxygen, and SAFFLOWER OIL: High in linoleic acid. nitrogen, and sometimes sulfur and phosphorus.

PUMPKIN: Enzymes in the whole "pumpkin", including the seeds, exfoliate dead skin cells while promoting skin repair. It cleanses, conditions and moisturizes while helping to firm the skin. Pumpkin is an excellent source of anti-oxidants, vitamins and essential elements the skin needs.

PUNICIC ACID- This acid is a conjugated linolenic acid or CLA; this means it has three (3) conjugated double bonds.

-Q-

QNATERNIUM-15 & 19: a preservative antimicrobial active against a wide spectrum of microorganisms. A quaternary ammonium salt.
QUATERNARY AMMONIUM SALTS (QUATS): Quaternium–7, 15, 31, 60, etc: This chemical breaks down in products into formaldehyde and causes the formation of carcinogenic nitrosamines under certain conditions.

-R-

RASPBERRY: Rich in minerals, ascorbic acid (vitamin C), flavonoids, tannins, and ellagic acid, a super antioxidant. Soothing, astringent and exfoliating. Percentage of AHAs: 10 citric, 5 glycolic, 8malic, 2 lactic.

RAW CANE SUGAR: Rich in "natural" glycolic acids, it has cellular renewal properties. Raw sugar cane is particularly rich in mucilage, thus being softening and moisturizing to the skin. Percentage AHAs: 2.5 citric, 15 glycolic, 2.5malic, 5 lactic.

REDUCING AGENT: Reducing agents are ingredients which during their reaction with oxidizing agents lose electrons. Reducing agents commonly contribute hydrogen to other substances. They can be used as antioxidants since they scavenge oxygen. In addition, reducing agents have the ability to split disulfide bonds in hair.

RETINYL PALMITATE: Vitamin A; a primary anti-oxidant, free radical scavenger and cell renewal ingredient.

RICE BRAN OIL: Rich in vitamin E. It has a smaller molecule than wheat germ oil making it much easier to penetrate the skin. Contains high percentages of oleic, linoleic and linolenic acids.

ROSEHIPS: The fruit of the rose bush, high in vitamin C; tonic, astringent, soothing to the skin.

ROSEMARY: Cleansing, anti-bacterial, anti-fungal, moisturizing, softening, rejuvenating.

-S-

SAFFLOWER OIL: High in linoleic acid.

SAGE: is a very effective herb for weak hair. is also effective for dark brown or black hair Spicy scent, effective for skin disruptions, treats hair imbalance. Antiseptic and stimulates circulation. It has a tautening effect making it ideal for aging skin.

SALICYLIC ACID: Occurs naturally in wintergreen leaves, sweet birch and other plants. Topically it is an anesthetic, a sunscreen and a fungicide with a mild peeling effect.

SAPONIFICATION: A another name for sop. It is the result amid a caustic alkali (lye) and fatty acids found in vegetable oil or animal fat.

SAW PALMETTO: This herb best used in powder form is known to help hair growth in women. Its anti-DHT ingredients include saw palmetto, Azealiic acid, and panthenol, all of which block DHT receptors in the hair follicles, which allows for hair growth

SEA ALGAE EXTRACT: A purified and recombined fractionation of Hawaiian sea plants. It is an excellent moisturizer that is extracted without the use of harsh chemicals.

SEA ALGAE/SEA KELP: See ALGAE.

SEA BUCKTHORN: Grows on the sand dunes by the sea and produces a yellow berry. The liquid wax from the berry is very compatible with the lipid structure of the skin and provides strong water retentive and skin moisturizing qualities.

SEA PALM: Very rich in potassium, beta-carotenoids, and a wealth of co-enzymes and trace minerals. It is known as the most elastic of all seaweeds and used as a connective tissue enhancer.

SEAWEED ESSENTIAL OIL: A CO-2 microburst extraction of French kelp varieties of seaweed; it yields aromatic oil and the protoplasmic bio-substance of the ocean to help open the capillaries in the skin's tissues bringing up much needed nutrients and oxygen from deep within the skin.

SHEA BUTTER: Shea butter is an emollient. It is extremely therapeutic, helping to heal cracked, aged and damaged skin. Shea butter penetrates the skin and leaves it feeling soft and smooth. It has vitamin A, E and is highly compatible with skin. Shea butter has a high content of unsaponifiables and cinnamic esters, which have antimicrobial and moisturizing properties and provide protection from the UV rays of the sun.

SLIP MODIFIER: Ingredients that help other substances to flow more easily and more smoothly, without reacting chemically.

SOAP BARK: Healing properties, emulsifier.

SODIUM LAUREL or (Lauryl) Sulfate (SLS) / Sodium Laureth Sulfate (SLES): This harsh detergent is found in car washes, engine degreasers, and garage floor cleaners as well as in over 90% of the personal care products. It is used for its foaming action. It causes eye irritations, skin rashes and allergic reactions. SLS breaks down the skin's moisture barrier and easily penetrates the skin allowing other chemicals to easily penetrate the skin as well. When combined with other chemicals, SLS can be transformed into "nitrosamines", a potent class of carcinogens. The American Journal of Toxicology states that SLS stays in the body up to 5 days. Sodium Lauryl Sulfate is frequently disguised in pseudo-natural personal care products as "comes from coconut". It is believed to cause hair loss and scalp irritation similar to dandruff.

SOLVENT: Substances, usually liquids, that are used to dissolve other substances.

SORBITOL: With a velvet soft feel to the skin this ingredient comes from apples, cherries, berries, plums, pears, sea algae and seaweed. Acts as an humectant, emulsifier and thickener in formulations.

SOYBEAN OIL: Rich in fatty acids and vitamin E; readily absorbs into the skin.

SQUALANE: An exquisite natural oil derived from olives, that moisturizes the skin and helps enhance skin's natural barrier function. Protects the skin against the elements and boosts the skin's ability to retain moisture. It is a natural bactericide and healer.

SUNFLOWER OIL: This carrier oil is extracted from the seeds of the sunflower. It is loaded with Linoleic acid and vitamins A, B Complex, D and E This oil helps to heal lubricate and moisturize the skin. This oil is considered an Emollient. It is known to have calcium, zinc, potassium, iron, and phosphorus.

SURFACTANT: An ingredient that helps two opposite substances mix, it allows the ingredients to become dissolved or evenly distributed in one another. Can be considered as a surface active agent.

- **CLEANSING AGENT:** Surfactants that clean skin and hair by helping water to mix with oil and dirt so that they can be rinsed away.
- **EMULSIFYING AGENT**: Surfactants that help to form emulsions by reducing the surface tension of the substances to be emulsified.
- **FOAM BOOSTER-** Surfactants that increase foaming capacity or that stabilize foams.
- **HYDROTROPE:** Surfactants that have the ability to enhance the water solubility of another surfactant.
- **SOLUBILIZING AGENT:** Surfactants that help another ingredient to dissolve in a solvent in which it would not normally dissolve

STEARIC ACID: (Vegetable). A white, waxy, fatty acid used as an emulsifying agent. Derived from vegetable fatty acids; soothes, softens and is an emulsifier.

STEARALKONIUM CHLORIDE: This chemical is used in hair conditioners and creams. It can cause allergic reactions. It was developed by the fabric industry as a fabric softener and is much cheaper and easier to use in hair conditioning formulae than proteins and herbals. It is considered toxic.

STRAWBERRY: Soothing, astringent, and firming; strawberries contain more vitamin C than an orange and also contains ellagic acid, a super antioxidant.

SWEET ALMOND OIL: Excellent emollient high in oleic, linoleic and other fatty acids, ideal in the treatment of very dry skin. Soothing and moisturizing. A good absorption base. The kernel of the almond is a very effective moisturizer for the skin and hair.

-T-

TAMARIND: Is a large evergreen tree that grows in the tropics. Percentage of AHAs: 10 citric, 5 malic, 10 tartaric.

TANNIN ACID: An astringent vegetable product found in a wide variety of plants. Sources include the bark of oak, hemlock, chestnut, and mangrove; the leaves of certain sumacs; and plant galls.

TEA TREE OIL: (Melaleuca alternifolia). From the leaves of the Australian tea tree, this oil is used to treat acne, cuts, burns, insect bites, fungus and other skin and scalp disorders. Oily hair. Treatment for dry scalp, dandruff, lice, and underactive sebaceous glands.

TIME RELEASE LIPOSOME COMPLEX: A range of vitamin and herbal phyto-active supplements to be time delivered into the skin for a continuous gentle release of vital nutrients.

TITANIUM DIOXIDE: A natural white powder mineral with the distinction of being a class one, full spectrum sunscreen. In cosmetic use it has the greatest concealing power of all white pigments.

TOCOPHEOL: Vitamin E. An anti-oxidant and cellular renewal ingredient that when combined with vitamins A and C, acts as a preservative in the oil phase of cosmetic formulations.

TOMATO: See Lycopene.

THYME: Anti-microbial and anti-inflammatory with astringent properties that help firm collagen in the skin.

-U-

ULTRAMARINE BLUE: An inorganic, FDA-approved, high-purity pigment

ULTRAMARINE PINK: An inorganic, FDA-approved, high-purity pigment

ULTRAMARINE VIOLET: An inorganic, FDA-approved, high-purity pigment

ULVA: A sea plant known as "sea lettuce" because of its bright green lettuce like leaf; a high source of soluble iron, potassium, and complex polysaccharides compatible with natural skin oils.

UVA URSI: Bearberry (or manzanita). It is the astringency of the tannin acid on the berries and leaves of this plant that make them work well as a natural source of hydroquinone (pigment lightener).

-V-

Vitamin A: (Beta Carotene) Helps maintain smooth, soft disease-free skin; helps protect the mucous membranes of the mouth, nose, throat lungs, which helps reduce our susceptibility to infections; protects against air pollutants and contaminants; helps improve eye sight and counteracts night-blindness; aids in bone and teeth formation; improves skin elasticity, moisture content and suppleness; and helps reverse the signs of photo-aging. A lack of vitamin A can cause skin to become dry and hardened.

Vitamin B5: Pantothenic Acid: Participates in the release of energy from carbohydrates, fats & protein, aids in the utilization of vitamins; improves the body's resistance to stress; helps in cell building & the development of the central nervous system; helps the adrenal glands, fights infections by building antibodies.

Vitamin C (Ascorbic Acid) : Vitamin C essential for healthy teeth, gums and bones. Helps to heal wounds, scar tissue, fractures; prevents scurvy; builds resistance to infection; aids in the prevention treatment of the common cold; gives strength to blood vessels; aids in the absorption of iron. It is required for the synthesis of collagen, the intercellular cement which holds tissues together. It is also one of the major antioxidant nutrients. It prevents the conversion of nitrates (from tobacco smoke, smog, bacon, lunchmeats, some vegetables) into cancer-causing substances. Moreover, Vitamin C has been shown to help slow the production of hyperpigmentation (age spots) while providing some UV protection.

Vitamin E: Vitamin E is a major anti-oxidant nutrient that retards cellular aging due to oxidation; supplies oxygen to the blood which is then carried to the heart and other organs; thus alleviating fatigue; aids in bringing nourishment to cells; strengthens the capillary walls prevents the red blood cells from destructive poisons; prevents dissolves blood clots; has also been used by doctors in helping prevent sterility, muscular dystrophy, calcium deposits in blood walls and heart conditions.

WHEAT GERM OIL: A natural source of vitamins A, E and D, and squalene.

-W-

WHEAT PROTEIN: A highly refined, natural protein derived from whole wheat. Wheat protein improves body and shine while imparting conditioned feel to the hair.

WILLOW BARK: A source of salicin, the chemical that led to the introduction of aspirin, considered to be the natural form and origin of the modern day aspirin. An anti-inflammatory agent delivered to the skin cells in liposomes that enhance penetration through the epidermis. Causes a mild keratolytic effect making it an excellent ingredient for acne treatment products.

WITCH HAZEL: improves skin tone, helps restore circulation and fights broken capillaries. This herb works as a astringent and is great for tired, sluggish, oily, dry, and infected skin. A natural astringent known for shrinking skin pores.

-X-

XANTHAN GUM: A natural carbohydrate gum used as a thickener and emulsion stabilizer.

-Y-

YARROW: Moisturizing, softening, and soothing with mild astringency.

YEAST: A calming extract. When combined with glycosaminoglycans and glycopolysaccarides. They help:

1. Increase superficial and deep skin firmness.
2. Increase collagen synthesis and reduce wrinkles.
3. Increase moisture.
4. Increase skin clarity

YLANG-YLANG OIL: A natural antiseptic essential oil with soothing properties.

YUCCA: Cleansing, soothing. a wetting agent which contributes to skin soothing and healing.

-Z-

ZINC: A natural mineral. Calming, with osmosis and diffusion qualities.

ZINC OXIDE: A natural "skin protecting" sunscreen agent; antiseptic, and astringent.

REFERENCES

- Hess WM, Seegmiller RE, Gardner JS, Allen JV, Barendregt S. Human hair morphology: a scanning electron microscopy study on a male Caucasoid and a computerized classification of regional differences. Scanning Microsc. 1990 Jun;4(2):375-86.
- Dawber RP. An update of hair shaft disorders. Dermatol Clin. 1996 Oct;14(4):753-72.
- Caserio RJ. Diagnostic techniques for hair disorders. Part I: Microscopic examination of the hair shaft. Cutis. 1987 Sep;40(3):265-70.
- Caserio RJ. Diagnostic techniques for hair disorders. Part II: Microscopic examination of hair bulbs, tips, and casts. Cutis. 1987 Oct;40(4):321-5.
- Rogers M. Hair shaft abnormalities: Part I. Australas J Dermatol. 1995 Nov;36(4):179-84; quiz 185-6.
- Rogers M. Hair shaft abnormalities: Part II. Australas J Dermatol. 1996 Feb;37(1):1-11.
- Whiting DA. Structural abnormalities of the hair shaft. J Am Acad Dermatol. 1987 Jan;16(1 Pt 1):1-25.
- Hutchinson PE. Diagnosis of hair disease. Practitioner. 1980 Nov;224(1349):1159-67.
- Crounse RG. The diagnostic value of microscopic examination of human hair. Arch Pathol Lab Med. 1987 Aug;111(8):700-2.
- Shelley WB. Hair examination using double-stick tape. J Am Acad Dermatol. 1983 Mar;8(3):430-1.
- Bottoms E, Wyatt E, Comaish S. Progressive changes in cuticular pattern along the shafts of human hair as seen by scanning electron microscopy. Br J Dermatol. 1972 Apr;86(4):379-84.
- Dawber R, Comaish S. Scanning electron microscopy of normal and abnormal hair shafts. Arch Dermatol. 1970 Mar;101(3):316-22.
- Caputo R, Ceccarelli B. Study of normal hair and of some malformations with a scanning electron microscope. Arch Klin Exp Dermatol. 1969;234(3):242-9.
- Nikiforidis G, Balas C, Tsambaos D. Mechanical parameters of human hair: possible application in the diagnosis and follow-up of hair disorders. Clin Phys Physiol Meas. 1992 Aug;13(3):281-90.
- Niyogi SK. Abnormality of hair shaft due to disease. Its forensic importance. J Forensic Med. 1968 Oct-Dec;15(4):148-51

WEBSITES

www.naturallycurly.com/texture-typing/hair-porosity
www.keratin.com/
www.andrewalkerhair.com
www.dadamo.com
www.calvizie.net/documento.asp?args=7.1.414

GLOSSARY REFERENCES:

- http://www.simplydivinebotanicals.com/findusnearyou.html
- http://www.melangecosmetics.com/ingredients.htm

SANITATION & STERILIZATION:

- https://quizlet.com/20152019/chapter-05-infection-control-miladys-standard-esthetics-flash-cards/
- http://www.clive.canoe.ca/Health9906/07_linton.html
- http://www.chumd.com/LifeStyle/Personal_Health/12-NOV-2000/102901_en.html
- http://www.epa.gov/region4/
- Milady Textbook of Cosmetology The Van Dean Manual http://www.salonsafety.com/safetysheets
- http://www.dca.ca.gov/barber/barbcmpl.htm
- http://medicalreporter.health.org/tmr0499/hair_and_nail_salons_linked_to_i.htm
- http://www.doctormercola.com/personal-hygiene/get-beautiful-lustrous-hair-with-coconut-oil/

ARTICLES

- Natural Health Articles by Dr. Joseph Mercola Coconut Oil…

INFECTIOUS HAIR DISEASE REFERENCES

- Roberts BJ, Friedlander SF. Tinea capitis: a treatment update. Pediatr Ann. 2005 Mar;34(3):191-200. PMID: 15792111
- Kyle AA, Dahl MV. Topical therapy for fungal infections. Am J Clin Dermatol. 2004;5(6):443-51. PMID: 15663341
- Luelmo-Aguilar J, Santandreu MS. Folliculitis: recognition and management. Am J Clin Dermatol. 2004;5(5):301-10. PMID: 15554731
- Gupta AK, Batra R, Bluhm R, Boekhout T, Dawson TL Jr. Skin diseases associated with Malassezia species. J Am Acad Dermatol. 2004 Nov;51(5):785-98. PMID: 15523360
- Guay DR. Treatment of bacterial skin and skin structure infections. Expert Opin Pharmacother. 2003 Aug;4(8):1259-75. PMID: 12877635
- Hainer BL. Dermatophyte infections. Am Fam Physician. 2003 Jan 1;67(1):101-8. PMID: 12537173
- Stulberg DL, Penrod MA, Blatny RA. Common bacterial skin infections. Am Fam Physician. 2002 Jul 1;66(1):119-24. PMID: 12126026
- Mengesha YM, Bennett ML. Pustular skin disorders: diagnosis and treatment. Am J Clin Dermatol. 2002;3(6):389-400. PMID: 12113648
- Gupta AK, Summerbell RC. Tinea capitis. Med Mycol. 2000 Aug;38(4):255-87. Review. PMID: 10975696
- Weitzman I, Summerbell RC. The dermatophytes. Clin Microbiol Rev. 1995 Apr;8(2):240-59. PMID: 7621400

HAIR COLOR - WHAT IS IT REFERENCES

- Commo S, Bernard BA. Melanocyte subpopulation turnover during the human hair cycle: an immunohistochemical study. Pigment Cell Res. 2000 Aug;13(4):253-9.
- Tobin DJ, Slominski A, Botchkarev V, Paus R. The fate of hair follicle melanocytes during the hair growth cycle. J Investig Dermatol Symp Proc. 1999 Dec;4(3):323-32.
- Horikawa T, Norris DA, Johnson TW, Zekman T, Dunscomb N, Bennion SD, Jackson RL, Morelli JG. DOPA-negative melanocytes in the outer root sheath of human hair follicles express premelanosomal antigens but not a melanosomal antigen or the melanosome-associated glycoproteins tyrosinase, TRP-1, and TRP-2. J Invest Dermatol. 1996 Jan;106(1):28-35.
- Schallreuter K, Slominski A, Pawelek JM, Jimbow K, Gilchrest BA. What controls melanogenesis? Exp Dermatol. 1998 Aug;7(4):143-50.
- Tobin DJ, Hagen E, Botchkarev VA, Paus R. Do hair bulb melanocytes undergo apoptosis during hair follicle regression (catagen)? J Invest Dermatol. 1998 Dec;111(6):941-7.
- Slominski A, Paus R, Plonka P, Chakraborty A, Maurer M, Pruski D, Lukiewicz S. Melanogenesis during the anagen-catagen-telogen transformation of the murine hair cycle. J Invest Dermatol. 1994 Jun;102(6):862-9.
- Boissy RE and Nordlund JJ. Biology of melanocytes. In: Cutaneous Medicine and Surgery. Arndt KA, LeBoit PE, Robinson JK, and Wintroub BU, eds. W.B. Saunders Co: Philadelphia, 1996, pp.1203-1218. Slominski A, Paus R. Melanogenesis is coupled to murine anagen: toward new concepts for the role of melanocytes and the regulation of melanogenesis in hair growth. J Invest Dermatol. 1993 Jul;101(1 Suppl):90S-97S.

ALOPECIA AREATA OVERVIEW – REFERENCES

- Freyschmidt-Paul P, Happle R, McElwee KJ, Hoffmann R. Alopecia areata: treatment of today and tomorrow. J Investig Dermatol Symp Proc. 2003 Jun;8(1):12-7. PMID: 12894988
- McElwee KJ, Freyschmidt-Paul P, Sundberg JP, Hoffmann R. The pathogenesis of alopecia areata. J Investig Dermatol Symp Proc. 2003 Jun;8(1):6-11. PMID: 12894987
- McElwee KJ, Hoffmann R. Alopecia areata. Clin Exp Dermatol. 2002 Jul;27(5):410-7. PMID: 12190642
- Freyschmidt-Paul P, Hoffmann R, Levine E, Sundberg JP, Happle R, McElwee KJ. Current and potential agents for the treatment of alopecia areata. Curr Pharm Des. 2001 Feb;7(3):213-30. PMID: 11311114
- McElwee KJ, Tobin DJ, Bystryn JC, King LE Jr, Sundberg JP. Alopecia areata: an autoimmune disease? Exp Dermatol. 1999 Oct;8(5):371-9. PMID: 10536963

SCARRING ALOPECIAS REFERENCES

- Ross EK, Tan E, Shapiro J. Update on primary cicatricial alopecias. J Am Acad Dermatol. 2005 Jul;53(1):1-40. PMID: 15965418
- Tan E, Martinka M, Ball N, Shapiro J. Primary cicatricial alopecias: clinicopathology of 112 cases. J Am Acad Dermatol. 2004 Jan;50(1):25-32. PMID: 14699361
- Wiedemeyer K, Schill WB, Loser C. Diseases on hair follicles leading to hair loss part II: scarring alopecias. Skinmed. 2004 Sep-Oct;3(5):266-271. PMID: 15365263
- Olsen EA, Bergfeld WF, Cotsarelis G, Price VH, Shapiro J, Sinclair R, Solomon A, Sperling L, Stenn K, Whiting DA, Bernardo O, Bettencourt M, Bolduc C, Callendar V, Elston D, Hickman J, Ioffreda M, King L, Linzon C, McMichael A, Miller J, Mulinari F, Trancik R; Workshop on Cicatricial Alopecia. Summary of North American Hair Research Society (NAHRS)-sponsored Workshop on Cicatricial Alopecia, Duke University Medical Center, February 10 and 11, 2001. J Am Acad Dermatol. 2003 Jan;48(1):103-10. PMID: 12522378
- Headington JT. Cicatricial alopecia. Dermatol Clin. 1996 Oct;14(4):773-82. PMID: 9238335

CLUB HAIR REFERENCES

- Headington JT. Telogen effluvium. New concepts and review. Arch Dermatol. 1993 Mar;129(3):356-63.
- Sperling LC. Hair anatomy for the clinician. J Am Acad Dermatol. 1991 Jul;25(1 Pt 1):1-17.
- Ebling FJ. The biology of hair. Dermatol Clin. 1987 Jul;5(3):467-81.

TELOGEN EFFLUVIUM REFERENCES

- Rebora A. Telogen effluvium. Dermatology. 1997;195(3):209-12.
- Headington JT. Telogen effluvium. New concepts and review. Arch Dermatol. 1993 Mar;129(3):356-63.
- Guarrera M, Rebora A. Anagen hairs may fail to replace telogen hairs in early androgenic female alopecia. Dermatology. 1996;192(1):28-31.
- Camacho F, Moreno JC, Garcia-Hernandez MJ. Telogen alopecia from UV rays. Arch Dermatol. 1996 Nov;132(11):1398-9.
- Rebora A. Telogen effluvium: an etiopathogenetic theory. Int J Dermatol. 1993 May;32(5):339-40.
- Kligman AM. Pathologic dynamics of reversible hair loss in humans. I. Telogen effluvium. AMA Arch Dermatol. 1961;83: 175-98.
- Sulzberger MB, Witten VH, Kopf AW. Diffuse alopecia in women. AMA Arch Dermatol. 1960; 81:556-60

THANK YOU

I want to send several extraordinary thanks to people who have played a special role in my life:

To My Parents **Wyman and Maxine Frederick** for all your support:

> **Dadi** for the weekly phone calls to check up on me and my family for all the care and concern for me… for offering support that only Dadi (a Father) who truly love their children can offer. For being there for your grandchildren like they are Your first born… this Is why all your daughters still can call you Dadi- because you are the BEST DADI IN THE WORLD!!! I Love you…
> Thank You for loving us with all your heart mind and soul…We know,"that only the strong survive the weak fall by wayside" your favorite quote…
>
> To **Momi**, I have come to love you more than you would ever know. You have been the one to keep us lifted up in prayer in your prayer closet, I'm sure your prayer room would be just like the movie- there would notes upon notes, letters upon letters posted up all over the walls from the floor to the roof in your prayer closet as it concerned your children life family and others and the best part of this all would be all the answered prayers at that. You have been faithful and because of this we call you BLESSED.
> As the oldest daughter who had two sisters looking up to her I secretly looked up to you. For your strength, integrity and prayer life. Because of the grace of GOD, You, have made us the women (daughters) we are today…I LOVE YOU. and hope every day you know it, you sense it and that you believe it…we too still call you MOMI 'cause, there is no Momi like our Momi and like we say when we are in difficult situations or trying to get each other right

or to shut each other up all we have to say is…. "Mom Said"…that's it & that's all she wrote- because we know you speak truth from the WORD of GOD!!!!

To a Woman of GOD who really would not even want to be acknowledged:
I extol you, I love you with all my heart ***Rose Reid*** my first other mother who was there with me when I began this Holistic journey. You were with me before the beginning of all of this. You were the shoulder I leaned on, the Godly ear that I needed. You remained here unconditionally with me through all my ups downs, the tears that I cried as a young wife and mother -you encouraged me, prayed with me and kept me lifted up before GOD the entire time. You were one of my first clients who would test all my products, and you have encouraged me throughout the years and I so appreciate you, love you and miss our time together.

To my Spiritual Parents for all your Dedicated Godly spiritual guidance and support:
Pastor Billy (Dad) you are indeed a true man of worship who is richly endowed with integrity. You walk in a Genuine Godly love that only a true God-ordained Apostle/pastor that sincerely LOVEs GOD can offer. I want to personally say Thank You for believing in me and the gifts that GOD has placed in me. I appreciate all the many hours of prayer praise and worship that you have labored before GOD on our behalf, and for the souls the many souls that has a true authentic burden in your life. May you continue to evolve in all that GOD has for you and be bless beyond measure. Lastly, like you say often- I will follow you as you continue to follow Christ and you do this effortlessly…Love you Pastor Billy

Prophet Cynthia (Mom) the labor of love cannot be truly expressed in these few sentences, you give relentlessly, your pour out continually, you prophesy uncompromisingly all with the heart and love and mind of GOD. Thank you for excepting me for me and for believing in me when I didn't even know or understand all that GOD had for me. You recognized things in me that I was not aware of and ascribe to even today. Love oozes from you with a hug, a phone call, a wave or even a simple, "Hello how are you doing"…the presence of God is so tangible and real in your life. Your global presence changes atmospheres that causes people lives to shift and allows generational things to be displaced, your prayer life is an example laid out before us to follow. It's a privileged and an honor to have you in my life and apart of this journey. I appreciate you so much. May GOD continually bless you and increase you and Pastor Billy and grant you all the desires of your heart. I dearly Love you as my Spiritual Mom and Godly Mentor.

To my other Spiritual Mom **Apostle Alice J Jones**
To one of most Special Woman I have ever had the pleasure to meet Apostle Alice J. Jones, you came into my life at one of lowest point a person could be at. We spent one day because of the leading of the Holy Spirit and I truly apologize now for talking your ears off…you sat and listened and heard everything I had to say and with a soft gentle voice hours later- you assured me… "it's going to be alright" soon after you became my Naomi and I became your Ruth…and we have been together ever since. I thank you for all the conversations, prayers, laughter and love that we have shared and will continue to share. As you aspire to reach deeper depths and higher heights in Him may GOD continue to keep you and Bless more and more Love you-Mom

Another Jewel God Blessed me with I offer up great Appreciation for is **Prophet Maureen Wray**:

I call you Mom Wray because you deserve to be distinguished as such, you took me & my family under your care like your own children, you have been with me for the long haul as well, all the times you would come over and I would do your hair and nothing but the wisdom of GOD and ministry would go forth and with it came the blessings that at that time in my life my family's life was so needed. Thank you for your many, many prayers and intercessor lifestyle that precedes you…thank you for being there for me and with me and also for my family…I can't say thank you enough…you are so needed and necessary in the body of Christ…I love you so much Mom Wray ☺

I send a great word of Acknowledgement to one of my Big Sisters who is also a Giant in Christ, Anointed and Awesome in her own right **Minister Darshane Harris**

Silently you have been the wind beneath my wings, with all the calls of love, concern and encouragement. Every prayer that you have prayed with me and words of life spoken over me to help the process become a little easier. You as well have believed in me spoke life to me and offered me and my family nothing but the love of GOD. I truly thank you I pray that you walk in and attain ALL that GOD has for you NOW in this lifetime.

To my sisters and brother **Wyman, Jr, Robin Lightbourn, Angela Collie**: I can't say enough about y'all.. people look at us and wonder how can we be this close, in Helen Baylor voice… (We have a praying Mother)!!!!. We talk every day if not every other day- we pray together, laugh together, get mad and get over it together… I could not have asked for a better set of siblings than the ones GOD so blessed me with…and although y'all didn't speak for me at my first seminar (it made me better) LOL… I love y'all even more for this. We are on top and rising for the Glory of GOD.

I can't and won't forget my Bestie my girl of all these years **Aijalonne Bookker**:

Girl you got my back you have been ride or die chick and although we don't spend a lot of time together it's like there is no love or time lost when we meet up and talk. Thank you for the care love and concern for me and my family. I acknowledge you because you are beautiful inside and out and it's hard to find friend like this. I treasure our friendship more than you know…keep reaching for the best because you deserve it and more… Love you girl!!!!

And lastly my brother from my other mother…**Michael Harris-** Thank you for all the inspiration to continue to go forward with my company, product line and this book, you have checked up on me throughout my physical challenges and offered insight on proper exercise and so on…it's the little things that were so helpful…it's the conversations that you have had with me & Lij over dinner or just sitting around the house… from the first evening we met and talked until your flight at 6 AM. IN THE MORNING!!!!!... we have been inseparable it's like we have known each other since children. I appreciate YOU, your wisdom, knowledge, insight and conversations. Now may all that you put your hands to continue to prosper and bring GOD all the Glory stay on top and keep rising…Love you Bro.

ABOUT THE AUTHOR

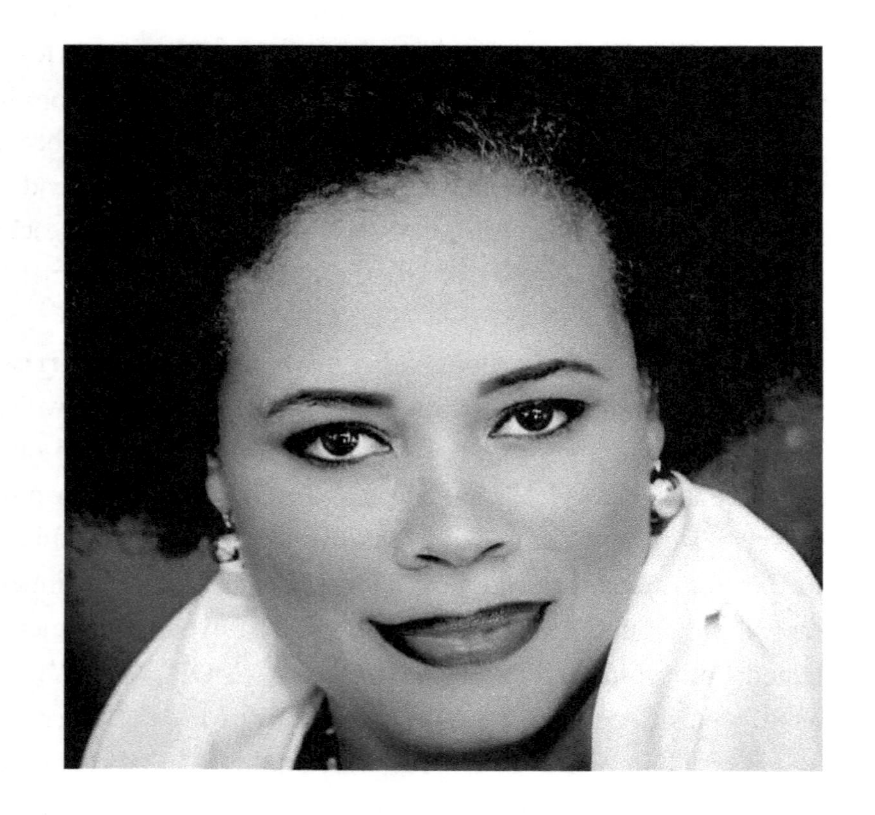

PAMELA FREDERICK MAIR

Pamela Frederick Mair is the Owner, CEO and Founder of Rxestoratives Hair and Skin Wellness® Inc., where she is a Holistic Cosmetologist, Hair Health Coach, Educator, Nutritional Consultant and the manufacturer of an all-natural hair & skin product line. Pamela is the wife of Lij M. Mair Sr., a mother of two children, and a grandmother of two as well.

Pamela's mission is to teach consumers how to have "Healthy Hair at Home." As a Licensed Holistic Cosmetologist, and a Holistic Nutritional Consultant, Pamela is committed to providing a safe, supportive and empowering environment best suited for your hair, body and skin care needs. Pamela offers Holistic Nutritional Consultations, and seminars with insightful guidance to gain a deeper understanding of how to maintain optimal health and vitality for your hair, body, and skin.

Pamela's believes "what goes in is what comes out!" Once the consumer has a full understanding of the concept of healing, health and wellness; restoration is within reach.

As a specialty consultant, Pamela creates an effective holistic hair and skin régime according to the clients, specific needs and goals. She states, "Our body has the God given natural ability to heal itself" in which she strongly believes. She provides gentle guidance to aid in the healing and restorative process, whether it's for your body or the overall health of your hair and skin.

Nutrition is one of the key factors in attaining optimal overall health. Through a verbal, visual evaluation, and a written assessment of your current diet and lifestyle, a nutritional program can be tailored to meet your specific needs. It's her goal for you to construct a healthier, happier, and balanced life style for optimal health and beautiful skin and to have stronger longer thicker hair. At her practice, Pamela's ability is to manufacture specific all natural products just for you which, will facilitate a beautiful transformation to a healthy overall lifestyle. With a full understanding of the proper use of products, ingredients, food, vitamins, and knowing the required applications for hair and skin product; YOU CAN HAVE HEALTHY HAIR AT HOME!